AF836240

Food Deserts

Inequality in Nutrition

Mark Evans

ISBN: 978-1-77890-486-8
Imprint: darkside.exe
Copyright © 2024 Mark Evans.
All Rights Reserved.

Contents

Introduction to Food Deserts

Definition and Explanation

Defining food deserts

In order to understand the concept of food deserts, it is important to first define what exactly constitutes a food desert. A food desert is typically defined as an area where residents have limited access to affordable and nutritious food, particularly fresh fruits and vegetables. These areas are often characterized by the absence of full-service grocery stores within a reasonable distance. Instead, residents may rely on convenience stores or fast food restaurants, which typically offer limited healthy food options.

There are several key components that contribute to the definition of a food desert. Firstly, the distance to a full-service grocery store is a crucial factor. In urban areas, a commonly used measure is the distance to the nearest grocery store, with a threshold of one mile often used to designate an area as a food desert. In rural areas, where distances are larger, the threshold is usually increased to ten miles.

Secondly, the availability of transportation in these areas is important. Even if a full-service grocery store is located within a reasonable distance, if residents do not have access to reliable transportation, their ability to access nutritious food is severely limited. Lack of access to private vehicles and infrequent or unreliable public transportation can exacerbate the issue of food deserts.

Thirdly, the affordability of healthy food is a significant factor in determining whether an area is a food desert. Even if a grocery store is accessible, if the prices of fresh fruits, vegetables, and other nutritious food items are exorbitantly high, it can deter low-income individuals and families from purchasing these items. This can lead to a reliance on cheaper, but less nutritious, processed and fast foods.

It is important to note that the definition of a food desert is not limited to geographic factors alone. Socioeconomic and demographic characteristics of an area also play a role. Low-income neighborhoods, where residents may have limited financial resources to access healthy food options, are more likely to be classified as food deserts. Additionally, areas with high concentrations of poverty, racial and ethnic minorities, and limited educational opportunities are disproportionately affected by food deserts.

Food deserts can have serious implications for the health and well-being of individuals residing in these areas. Limited access to fresh and nutritious food can result in a diet that is high in processed foods, which are often calorie-dense but nutrient-poor. This can contribute to a range of health issues, including obesity, diabetes, cardiovascular disease, and other diet-related chronic conditions.

In recent years, efforts have been made to address the issue of food deserts through various interventions and policies. This includes initiatives aimed at improving access to healthy food options, such as the establishment of farmers markets, community gardens, and mobile food markets. Furthermore, policy changes have been implemented to incentivize grocery stores to open in underserved areas and provide affordable and nutritious food options.

In conclusion, food deserts are areas where residents have limited access to affordable and nutritious food. Factors such as distance to grocery stores, availability of transportation, affordability of healthy food, and socioeconomic and demographic characteristics contribute to the definition of food deserts. The impacts of food deserts on health are significant, leading to a higher prevalence of diet-related chronic diseases. Efforts are being made to address this issue through various interventions and policies aimed at improving access to healthy food options in underserved areas.

Factors contributing to food deserts

Food deserts are areas with limited access to affordable and nutritious food, often found in low-income communities. Several factors contribute to the emergence and persistence of food deserts, exacerbating inequalities in nutrition. Understanding these factors is crucial for developing effective interventions and policies to address this issue.

1. Economic Factors: Socioeconomic status plays a significant role in the existence of food deserts. High poverty rates and low median incomes in certain neighborhoods make it financially unviable for grocery stores and supermarkets to operate. The lack of demand, combined with high operational costs, deters businesses from investing in these areas, leading to limited availability of fresh and healthy food options.

2. Neighborhood Demographics: The racial and ethnic composition of a neighborhood can affect the presence of food deserts. Historically marginalized communities, such as those predominantly African American or Hispanic, are disproportionately affected by food deserts. Discrimination and structural inequalities have limited access to financial resources and opportunities, contributing to the perpetuation of food deserts in these areas.

3. Physical Infrastructure: The spatial distribution and layout of neighborhoods can contribute to food deserts. In urban areas, the absence of grocery stores and supermarkets is particularly prevalent in areas with a high population density and limited available land. Conversely, rural areas face challenges related to the distance between communities and stores, as well as inadequate transportation infrastructure.

4. Transportation Barriers: Lack of reliable and affordable transportation options can further exacerbate food deserts. Limited public transportation routes, especially in rural areas, make it difficult for residents to access stores with affordable and nutritious food. Additionally, the high cost of private transportation can be a barrier for low-income individuals, making it challenging to travel to stores located outside their neighborhoods.

5. Food Retail Environment: The nature of the food retail environment within a neighborhood can contribute to the development of food deserts. Many low-income neighborhoods only have convenience stores or fast-food outlets that primarily offer processed and unhealthy food options. The lack of grocery stores with diverse and fresh food choices limits residents' ability to make healthier dietary choices.

6. Food System Dynamics: The overall food system impacts the existence of food deserts. Industrialized agriculture and the consolidation of food production and distribution have led to the dominance of large-scale supermarkets and grocery chains, which tend to locate in more affluent areas. This concentration of food retail excludes low-income communities, perpetuating food deserts.

7. Policy and Planning Decisions: Historical and contemporary policy decisions can contribute to the existence of food deserts. Zoning regulations, land use policies, and development decisions often prioritize commercial developments that cater to higher-income individuals. This results in the neglect of low-income neighborhoods, leading to limited access to quality food retailers.

Addressing these factors requires a multi-dimensional approach that encompasses both policy changes and community-based initiatives. Collaborative efforts involving government agencies, local communities, businesses, and advocacy organizations are essential for creating sustainable and equitable solutions to food deserts. By understanding the complex interactions and dynamics of the contributing factors, we can work towards building healthy and food-secure communities for all.

Explaining the impact of food deserts on nutrition

Food deserts, defined as areas with limited access to affordable and nutritious food, have a significant impact on the nutrition and health of individuals residing in these areas. In this section, we will explore the various ways in which food deserts affect nutrition and the implications for overall health and well-being.

Limited availability of fresh fruits and vegetables

One of the key consequences of living in a food desert is the limited availability of fresh fruits and vegetables. Grocery stores that offer a wide selection of fresh produce are often scarce in these areas, making it challenging for residents to incorporate these essential food items into their diet. As a result, individuals may rely heavily on processed and unhealthy foods that are more readily available, leading to poor nutrition and an increased risk of chronic diseases such as obesity, diabetes, and cardiovascular diseases.

Example: For instance, imagine a family living in a food desert where the nearest grocery store is miles away. They may not have access to fresh fruits and vegetables on a regular basis, and instead, resort to purchasing canned or frozen foods with lower nutritional value. This lack of access to fresh produce deprives them of essential vitamins, minerals, and dietary fiber, contributing to a suboptimal diet.

Higher prevalence of unhealthy food options

In addition to the limited availability of fresh produce, food deserts are often characterized by an overabundance of unhealthy food options, such as fast food restaurants, convenience stores, and corner shops. These establishments primarily offer highly processed and calorie-dense foods that are high in fats, sugars, and sodium. The ease of access and affordability of these options make them more appealing to residents, further exacerbating poor nutrition and contributing to the rise in obesity rates within food desert communities.

Example: Consider a low-income neighborhood with multiple fast food chains but no grocery store. The lack of healthier alternatives leaves residents with limited options for nourishing meals. Instead, they may regularly consume fast food meals that are high in calories and low in essential nutrients. These dietary patterns can lead to weight gain, nutrient deficiencies, and a higher risk of developing chronic diseases.

Cultural and socioeconomic factors

Food deserts are often associated with lower-income neighborhoods, where residents may face socioeconomic challenges that compound the impact on nutrition. Limited financial resources can make it difficult for individuals to afford healthier food options, as fresh produce and nutritious items are often more expensive than processed foods. Moreover, cultural factors, such as dietary preferences and food traditions, may play a role in shaping dietary choices within food deserts.

Example: Within a food desert community predominantly composed of low-income households with diverse cultural backgrounds, residents may rely on affordable and culturally familiar food options, which may not necessarily be nutritious. For instance, a family from a Hispanic background may consume processed snacks and sugary beverages due to their cultural significance or affordability, contributing to a less than optimal diet.

Impact on children and vulnerable populations

The impact of food deserts on nutrition is particularly significant for children and vulnerable populations, including pregnant women, older adults, and individuals with chronic illnesses. Inadequate access to nutritious foods can have long-lasting consequences on their growth, development, and overall health. Children growing up in food deserts are more likely to develop poor eating habits, experience slower growth, and face a higher risk of obesity and related health problems.

Example: Consider a food desert neighborhood with limited access to fresh fruits, vegetables, and other healthy food options. Pregnant women residing in this area may struggle to obtain essential nutrients, such as folate and iron, from their diet, leading to pregnancy complications and developmental issues in their unborn child. Similarly, older adults living in food deserts may be at a higher risk of malnutrition and age-related health problems due to the limited availability of nutritious meals.

Summary

The impact of food deserts on nutrition is multifaceted and extends beyond the limited availability of fresh produce. The prevalence of unhealthy food options, cultural and socioeconomic influences, and the disproportionate effect on vulnerable populations all contribute to poor nutrition and increased health risks within food desert communities. Addressing these challenges requires a comprehensive approach involving community-based initiatives, policy changes, and investments in improving access to affordable and nutritious food options. By recognizing the adverse impact of food deserts on nutrition, we can work towards creating equitable and healthier food environments for all individuals, regardless of their geographic location or socioeconomic status.

History and Origins of Food Deserts

The Emergence of Food Deserts

Food deserts have emerged as a critical issue in our modern society, exacerbating inequality in nutrition and impacting the health and well-being of communities. Understanding the emergence of food deserts requires a multidisciplinary approach, taking into account historical, sociological, and economic factors. This section delves into the origins and development of food deserts, shedding light on the complexities surrounding this phenomenon.

Historical Context and Societal Factors

The origins of food deserts can be traced back to various historical and societal factors. One key factor is urbanization, as large-scale migration from rural areas to cities during the Industrial Revolution resulted in the concentration of populations in urban centers. This shift led to the development of densely populated urban areas with inadequate access to fresh and healthy food.

Another influential factor is the rapid expansion of the food industry, particularly the rise of supermarkets and chain stores. This expansion was accompanied by a phenomenon known as "white flight," where wealthier white populations moved away from urban centers into suburban areas, leaving behind predominantly low-income and minority communities. As a result, supermarkets followed the affluent population, leaving inner-city neighborhoods without accessible grocery stores.

Additionally, economic disparities and income inequality have played a significant role in the emergence of food deserts. Low-income neighborhoods often lack the economic power to attract full-service grocery stores, which require substantial investment and demand higher profit margins. Consequently, these neighborhoods are left with limited and inadequate food retail options, such as convenience stores or fast food outlets, which offer predominantly unhealthy and processed foods.

Early Studies on Food Deserts

The emergence of food deserts as a research topic can be attributed to early studies conducted in the 1980s and 1990s. These seminal studies, such as those by Mari Gallagher and the United States Department of Agriculture, shed light on the geographic disparities in food access and the concentration of food insecurity in specific areas.

One notable study by Gallagher examined the supply and demand of food retailers in low-income neighborhoods of Chicago. She documented the disproportionate distribution of supermarkets and the prevalence of unhealthy food options in these areas. Gallagher's work sparked further research and ignited public awareness, leading to a growing understanding of the concept of food deserts.

The United States Department of Agriculture (USDA) has also played a crucial role in studying and addressing food deserts. Their research defines food deserts as areas with limited access to nutritious and affordable food, particularly those with low-income populations residing a certain distance from a full-service grocery store. The USDA's Food Access Research Atlas has been instrumental in identifying and mapping food deserts across the United States, providing a valuable resource for researchers and policymakers.

Exploring the Impact of Food Deserts

Understanding the impact of food deserts on nutrition is essential to comprehending the significance of this issue. Limited access to healthy food options has significant consequences for individuals and communities in food deserts.

Firstly, the absence of affordable fresh produce and nutritious food in food deserts contributes to dietary imbalances and the consumption of processed, high-calorie, and nutrient-poor foods. This unhealthy diet can lead to chronic health conditions such as obesity, diabetes, and heart disease. Consequently, individuals in food deserts are more vulnerable to nutrition-related health risks, further exacerbating health disparities.

Secondly, the lack of access to fresh and perishable foods inhibits the development of a balanced diet, particularly for vulnerable populations such as children and older adults. Nutritional deficiencies can have long-term consequences on physical and cognitive development in children, impacting their academic performance and overall well-being. Similarly, inadequate access to healthy food options can adversely affect the health and quality of life of older adults.

Furthermore, the limited food access in food deserts often forces residents to rely on unhealthy and expensive alternatives, such as fast food or convenience store staples. This reliance perpetuates a cycle of poor nutrition and exacerbates socioeconomic inequalities, as individuals in food deserts may allocate a significant portion of their income towards purchasing higher-priced and lower-quality food items.

It is essential to approach the issue of food deserts holistically, recognizing the intertwined social, economic, and health implications. By understanding the emergence of food deserts and their impacts, we can develop effective interventions and policies to address this pressing issue.

Summary

In this section, we explored the emergence of food deserts, considering historical, sociological, and economic factors. Urbanization, the expansion of the food industry, economic disparities, and income inequality have all contributed to the development of food deserts. Early studies on food deserts, including the seminal work of Mari Gallagher and the USDA, brought increased attention to the issue and highlighted the geographic disparities in food access. We also delved into the impact of food deserts on nutrition, emphasizing the health risks and socio-economic consequences associated with limited access to nutritious food. Understanding the origins and ramifications of food deserts is crucial for implementing effective interventions and advocating for positive change.

Historical Context and Societal Factors

To fully understand the emergence of food deserts, it is essential to examine the historical context and societal factors that have contributed to their development. This section will explore the key historical events and social dynamics that have shaped the landscape of food deserts.

Urbanization and the Rise of Food Deserts

The phenomenon of food deserts can be traced back to the rapid urbanization that took place in the 20th century. As populations shifted from rural areas to urban centers, there was a significant increase in the concentration of poverty and economic disparities in cities. This urbanization process led to the emergence of neighborhoods characterized by limited access to fresh, nutritious food, giving rise to what we now know as food deserts.

During the mid-20th century, urban planning and housing policies played a crucial role in perpetuating the unequal distribution of resources, including access to food. The development of low-income housing projects and the concentration of marginalized communities in specific areas further exacerbated the problem of food deserts. These communities were often located far away from grocery stores and supermarkets, with limited transportation options, making it difficult for residents to access healthy food.

Additionally, historical racial and ethnic segregation in cities has contributed significantly to the creation and persistence of food deserts. The discriminatory practices of redlining, where certain neighborhoods were systematically denied investment and resources based on their racial composition, resulted in the concentration of poverty and limited access to quality food in predominantly minority communities.

Disinvestment and the Decline of Inner Cities

Another critical factor that has contributed to the emergence of food deserts is the process of disinvestment in inner-city neighborhoods. As suburbs grew in popularity and richer populations moved away from the city centers, many urban areas experienced a decline in economic and social resources.

This disinvestment was driven by a variety of factors, including changing economic structures, deindustrialization, and the flight of businesses and jobs from urban areas. As a result, many inner-city neighborhoods were left with abandoned buildings, vacant lots, and a lack of basic amenities such as grocery stores. This disinvestment created a vicious cycle, as the absence of quality food options further deterred potential investments and perpetuated the existence of food deserts.

Structural Racism and Systemic Inequalities

The historical and ongoing presence of structural racism and systemic inequalities have played a significant role in shaping the landscape of food deserts. Communities of color, particularly African American and Hispanic communities, have been disproportionately affected by the lack of access to healthy food options.

Structural racism refers to the ways in which institutions and systems perpetuate racial inequalities, intentionally or unintentionally. In the case of food deserts, structural racism manifests through discriminatory practices such as redlining, as discussed earlier, which limited resources and opportunities in minority communities.

Systemic inequalities, including disparities in income, education, and employment opportunities, further contribute to the prevalence of food deserts. Minority communities often face higher levels of poverty and unemployment, making it difficult to afford and access healthy food. Limited educational opportunities in these communities also lead to a lack of nutrition knowledge and low health literacy, exacerbating the problem.

Historical Efforts to Address Food Deserts

Historically, addressing food deserts has been a complex and ongoing challenge. Recognizing the detrimental impact of limited access to healthy food on marginalized communities, various efforts have been made to mitigate the problem.

One notable example is the establishment of farmers markets and community gardens in food desert areas. These initiatives aim to provide fresh produce directly to community members while fostering a sense of community engagement and empowerment. By connecting local growers to consumers in food desert neighborhoods, these initiatives help alleviate some of the barriers to accessing nutritious food.

Policy changes have also been introduced to address the issue of food deserts. For instance, in the United States, the Healthy Food Financing Initiative (HFFI) was launched to provide financial support, tax incentives, and grants to stimulate the development of grocery stores and supermarkets in underserved areas. Similarly, some governments have implemented zoning regulations to encourage the establishment of grocery stores in food desert neighborhoods.

Despite these efforts, significant challenges remain in effectively combating food deserts. Issues such as transportation barriers, affordability of healthy food, and the institutional and structural barriers associated with systemic inequalities must be addressed comprehensively to create lasting change.

Conclusion

The historical context and societal factors surrounding food deserts are crucial in understanding their emergence and persistence. Urbanization, disinvestment, structural racism, and systemic inequalities have all contributed to the creation and perpetuation of food deserts.

Efforts to address this issue have included community-based approaches, policy changes, and technological solutions. While these interventions have shown promise, more comprehensive and sustained efforts are needed to ensure equitable access to healthy food for all individuals and communities.

In the next section, we will explore the current state of food deserts in the United States, focusing on their geographical distribution, demographic patterns, and prevalence in urban and rural areas. This understanding is essential for developing effective interventions to combat the issue of food deserts.

Early studies on food deserts

Early studies on food deserts played a crucial role in identifying and understanding the issues surrounding limited access to healthy food in underserved communities. These studies aimed to shed light on the factors contributing to food deserts and their impact on nutrition. In this section, we will explore the key findings and methodologies of some seminal studies on food deserts.

One of the pioneering studies in this field was conducted by the United States Department of Agriculture (USDA) in the 1990s. The study focused on urban areas and defined food deserts as neighborhoods with limited access to supermarkets or large grocery stores. The research emphasized the importance of these stores in providing affordable and healthy food options, especially fresh produce.

The USDA study used geographic mapping techniques to identify food deserts and analyze their prevalence across the United States. The researchers found that food deserts were more common in low-income areas, with a higher concentration of minority populations. This study highlighted the correlation between socioeconomic status, race, and the likelihood of living in a food desert.

Building on this research, another study led by Mari Gallagher in 2006 provided further insights into the problem of food deserts. Gallagher's study focused on the Chicago metropolitan area and employed a comprehensive approach to evaluate the impact of limited food access on health outcomes. The research team collected data on food store locations, health indicators, and demographic characteristics of different neighborhoods.

The study found a significant association between living in a food desert and increased rates of diet-related health problems, such as obesity and diabetes. Additionally, the research highlighted the disparities in food access based on race and income, with African American and low-income neighborhoods facing the highest levels of food insecurity.

To understand the underlying causes of food deserts, some early studies also explored the role of neighborhood characteristics and food environment. For example, a study conducted by Beaulac et al. in 2009 investigated how the food environment in various neighborhoods influenced residents' dietary behaviors. The researchers found that individuals living in areas with limited food access had poorer dietary patterns, consuming fewer fruits and vegetables and higher amounts of unhealthy processed foods.

Moreover, these early studies analyzed the impact of food deserts on multiple dimensions of well-being. For instance, a study by Dubowitz et al. in 2010 examined the association between neighborhood food environments and physical activity levels. The research showed that individuals living in food deserts were less likely to engage in regular physical activity, contributing to the overall sedentary lifestyle and health risks.

These studies laid the foundation for subsequent research on food deserts and underscored the urgency of addressing this issue to improve public health. The methodologies utilized in these early studies have been refined and replicated in various contexts to provide a comprehensive understanding of the complex factors contributing to food deserts.

It is important to note that while these early studies were instrumental in raising awareness about food deserts, they also faced certain limitations. One limitation is the reliance on self-reported data, which may introduce biases. Additionally, the focus on urban areas in many studies limited the understanding of food deserts in rural and remote regions.

In summary, early studies on food deserts played a crucial role in highlighting the disparities in food access and the detrimental effects on nutrition and health. These studies employed geographic mapping, data analysis, and comprehensive approaches to evaluate the impact of limited food access on diverse populations. The findings from these studies provided the groundwork for further research and interventions to address the challenges posed by food deserts.

Current State of Food Deserts in the United States

Geographical distribution of food deserts

Food deserts are areas where residents have limited access to affordable and nutritious food, particularly fresh fruits and vegetables. The geographical distribution of food deserts varies across different regions and neighborhoods, influenced by various factors such as population density, income levels, racial composition, and proximity to grocery stores. Understanding the spatial distribution of food deserts is crucial for identifying areas that are most affected by food insecurity and designing targeted interventions.

1.3.1.1 Population density and food deserts

One important factor that influences the geographical distribution of food deserts is population density. In densely populated urban areas, where there is a high concentration of residents, the demand for food is usually greater. As a result, there tends to be a higher number of grocery stores and food retailers, reducing the likelihood of food deserts. On the other hand, in sparsely populated rural areas, the population density is low, and the distance between households and grocery stores tends to be greater, increasing the likelihood of food deserts.

For example, in densely populated cities like New York City or Chicago, there may be a larger number of grocery stores and supermarkets per square mile, making food more accessible to residents. However, in rural areas like parts of Appalachia or the Midwest, where the population density is lower, residents may have to travel long distances to access a well-stocked grocery store.

1.3.1.2 Income levels and food deserts

Another critical factor in the geographical distribution of food deserts is income levels. Low-income neighborhoods are more likely to have limited access to affordable and nutritious food options. This can be due to the lack of grocery stores or supermarkets in these areas or the high prices of fresh produce in comparison to processed and unhealthy food options available at convenience stores.

Studies have shown that low-income neighborhoods and communities with a higher percentage of residents living below the poverty line are more likely to have food deserts. This is because grocery stores and supermarkets often locate in more affluent areas where residents have higher purchasing power and can afford to buy a variety of food options. The lack of affordable food choices in low-income neighborhoods contributes to disparities in nutrition and health outcomes.

For instance, in urban areas, low-income neighborhoods may have limited access to quality grocery stores, forcing residents to rely on small convenience stores or fast food restaurants for their food needs. These options often offer a limited selection of fresh and healthy foods, leading to poorer diets and higher rates of diet-related diseases.

1.3.1.3 Racial composition and food deserts

Historical and socio-cultural factors, including racial segregation and discrimination, also play a significant role in the distribution of food deserts. Studies have shown that minority communities, particularly African American and Hispanic populations, are more likely to reside in food deserts compared to predominantly white neighborhoods.

The legacy of racial discrimination, redlining, and urban disinvestment has led to the unequal distribution of resources, including grocery stores, in minority neighborhoods. This phenomenon, known as environmental racism, exacerbates health disparities and reinforces socioeconomic inequalities.

For example, in many inner-city neighborhoods with predominantly African American populations, there is a higher prevalence of food deserts. Limited access to quality food options contributes to higher rates of obesity, diabetes, and other diet-related health issues within these communities.

1.3.1.4 Proximity to grocery stores and food deserts

The distance between households and grocery stores also plays a crucial role in the geographical distribution of food deserts. Areas that are far away from supermarkets or grocery stores may be more likely to be designated as food deserts.

In urban areas, the proximity to grocery stores may vary significantly within a single city. Neighborhoods located in close proximity to central business districts or affluent areas are more likely to have easy access to well-stocked grocery stores. However, neighborhoods located in the outskirts or in low-income areas may lack adequate grocery options and may be classified as food deserts.

Similarly, in rural areas, the distance to the nearest grocery store or supermarket can be substantial. Residents may have to drive long distances to reach the closest grocery store, leading to limited food access and increased likelihood of food deserts.

1.3.1.5 Geographical variations in food deserts

The geographical distribution of food deserts is not uniform across the United States. There are regional differences and variations in the prevalence of food deserts, with some areas experiencing higher levels of food insecurity than others.

For example, research has shown that Southern states such as Mississippi, Alabama, and Louisiana have higher rates of food deserts compared to states in the Northeast or West Coast. These disparities can be attributed to factors such as poverty rates, racial composition, and access to transportation infrastructure.

Additionally, rural areas tend to have higher concentrations of food deserts compared to urban areas. Limited access to transportation, long distances to grocery stores, and economic challenges in rural communities contribute to higher levels of food insecurity.

In summary, the geographical distribution of food deserts is influenced by population density, income levels, racial composition, proximity to grocery stores, and regional variations. Understanding these spatial patterns is essential for implementing targeted interventions to address food insecurity and promote equitable access to nutritious food.

Urban vs. Rural Food Deserts

Food deserts can occur in both urban and rural areas, but there are distinct differences between the two. In this section, we will explore the characteristics of urban and rural food deserts, and discuss how these differences impact access to healthy and affordable food options.

Defining Urban and Rural Food Deserts

Urban food deserts refer to areas within cities or densely populated urban areas where residents have limited or no access to fresh and nutritious food. These areas are typically characterized by a lack of grocery stores or supermarkets that offer a wide selection of fresh produce, dairy products, and whole grains. Instead, residents often have to rely on convenience stores or fast food outlets, which tend to offer mostly processed and unhealthy foods.

On the other hand, rural food deserts are found in sparsely populated areas, typically far away from major cities or urban centers. In these areas, the lack of accessible transportation options and the long distances to the nearest grocery store make it difficult for residents to access healthy and affordable food. Additionally, the limited options for employment and economic opportunities in rural areas often contribute to the prevalence of food deserts.

Factors Contributing to Urban Food Deserts

The characteristics of urban areas, such as high population density and limited available land, contribute to the emergence of food deserts in cities. Some key factors that contribute to the existence of urban food deserts include:

- **Supermarket Redlining:** Supermarket redlining refers to the practice of grocery stores avoiding low-income urban neighborhoods, often due to perceived socioeconomic risks. This leads to a lack of full-service grocery stores in these areas, creating food deserts.

- **Gentrification:** Gentrification is the process of revitalizing urban neighborhoods, often resulting in the displacement of low-income residents. As wealthier residents move in, businesses catering to their preferences, such as trendy cafes or specialty stores, may replace traditional grocery stores, exacerbating food access issues for the remaining low-income residents.

- **Food Retail Concentration:** In some urban areas, there may be an overconcentration of unhealthy food options, such as fast food restaurants and corner stores that primarily sell processed foods. This can exacerbate the lack of access to fresh and nutritious foods in low-income neighborhoods.

Factors Contributing to Rural Food Deserts

Rural food deserts face unique challenges due to their remote locations and limited infrastructure. Some factors that contribute to the existence of rural food deserts include:

- **Geographical Barriers:** Rural areas often have limited road infrastructure and are located far away from major cities or towns. This creates longer travel distances to reach grocery stores, making it difficult for residents, particularly those without access to private transportation, to access healthy food options.

- **Market Size and Density:** The low population density in rural areas makes it economically unviable for grocery stores or supermarkets to establish and maintain operations. The small customer base combined with the higher costs of transportation and storage make it challenging for retailers to serve these areas.

- **Limited Agricultural Opportunities:** While rural areas may have abundant agricultural resources, economic and environmental factors can limit the availability of fresh and locally grown produce. Lack of access to agricultural resources, such as land, water, and capital, can restrict opportunities for local food production in rural communities.

Addressing Urban and Rural Food Deserts

Addressing urban and rural food deserts requires tailored strategies that consider the unique challenges faced by each. Some potential solutions include:

Urban Food Deserts:

- **Community-based Food Initiatives:** Engaging local communities in the development of community gardens, farmers markets, and urban farms can increase access to fresh produce in urban areas. These initiatives can also provide opportunities for education and empowerment, fostering a sense of community ownership over food resources.

- **Policy Interventions:** Implementing policies that incentivize full-service grocery stores to open in underserved urban neighborhoods can help alleviate food deserts. This can include tax incentives, grants, or zoning regulations that prioritize the establishment of grocery stores in low-income areas.

- **Mobile Markets and Food Delivery Services:** Utilizing mobile markets or food delivery services in urban areas can help mitigate the transportation barriers faced by residents. These innovative approaches bring fresh produce and nutritious food directly to the neighborhoods that need them most.

Rural Food Deserts:

- **Transportation Solutions:** Improving transportation infrastructure and providing affordable transportation options, such as shuttle services or mobile markets, can help rural residents access grocery stores located in nearby towns or cities.
- **Local Food Production:** Supporting local agriculture and facilitating access to farmland can help stimulate local food production in rural areas. This can be achieved through agricultural extension programs, land-use policies, and financial assistance for farmers.
- **Tech-Focused Solutions:** Utilizing technology, such as online grocery platforms and community-supported agriculture programs, can help bridge the gap between rural residents and quality food options. These platforms can facilitate the ordering and delivery of fresh produce directly to rural households.

In summary, urban and rural food deserts present distinct challenges in terms of access to healthy and affordable food. Understanding the factors contributing to food deserts in each context allows for the development of targeted interventions that can address the specific needs of urban and rural communities. By implementing a combination of policy changes, community-based initiatives, and innovative solutions, we can work towards reducing the prevalence of food deserts and creating healthier and more equitable food environments for all.

Demographics and Food Desert Prevalence

Understanding the demographics of areas affected by food deserts is crucial in addressing the problem and implementing effective solutions. In this section, we will explore the various demographic factors that contribute to the prevalence of food deserts and the implications they have on the affected populations.

Income Disparities and Food Desert Prevalence

Income disparities play a significant role in the prevalence of food deserts. Low-income communities often face greater challenges in accessing healthy and affordable food options. Limited financial resources can result in a reliance on cheap, processed, and unhealthy food that is readily available in food deserts.

Studies have consistently shown that low-income neighborhoods have a higher concentration of food deserts compared to areas with higher income levels. The lack of grocery stores and healthy food options in these areas perpetuates a cycle of poor nutrition and negative health outcomes, leading to a higher risk of chronic diseases such as obesity, diabetes, and cardiovascular diseases.

Example: In the city of St. Louis, Missouri, there is a significant disparity in income levels between neighborhoods. As a result, low-income areas like North St. Louis have a higher prevalence of food deserts, with limited access to fresh and nutritious food. This disparity contributes to health disparities and perpetuates the cycle of poverty and unhealthy eating habits.

Racial and Ethnic Disparities in Food Deserts

Racial and ethnic disparities are also closely linked to the prevalence of food deserts. African American and Hispanic communities, in particular, are disproportionately affected by limited access to healthy food options. This disparity can be attributed to various historical and socio-cultural factors, including systemic racism, discriminatory practices, and neighborhood segregation.

Studies have shown that predominantly African American and Hispanic neighborhoods have fewer supermarkets and grocery stores compared to predominantly white neighborhoods. This lack of access to fresh and healthy food reinforces existing health disparities, as these communities are more likely to experience higher rates of obesity, diabetes, and other diet-related diseases.

Example: Chicago's South Side, predominantly inhabited by African American communities, has been identified as a food desert. The limited presence of grocery stores and the abundance of fast food restaurants in the area contribute to higher rates of obesity and other health issues within the community.

Age and Food Desert Prevalence

The age distribution within a given area plays a role in the prevalence of food deserts. Some age groups, such as the elderly and children, are more vulnerable to the negative effects of limited food access.

Elderly Population: Older adults living in food deserts may face additional challenges due to limited mobility, health conditions, and financial constraints. These factors can exacerbate their vulnerability to inadequate nutrition and increase the risk of chronic diseases.

Children: The lack of access to nutritious food options in food deserts negatively impacts children's health and development. Proper nutrition during childhood is crucial for growth, cognitive development, and overall well-being. Food-insecure children are at a higher risk of physical and mental health problems, as well as poor academic performance.

Example: In rural areas of Appalachia, where poverty rates are high, both the elderly population and children suffer from limited access to healthy food. This lack of access contributes to higher rates of malnutrition, obesity, and other health issues within these vulnerable populations.

Gender Disparities and Food Desert Prevalence

While gender disparities may not directly influence food desert prevalence, they can exacerbate the impact of limited food access on certain populations. For instance, women who are heads of households or primary caregivers may face additional challenges in providing healthy meals for their families due to limited resources and time constraints.

Example: In low-income urban areas, single mothers may have to prioritize their limited financial resources towards other essential needs, such as housing and childcare, leaving little to no funds available for nutritious food. This financial strain further perpetuates the cycle of food insecurity and poor health outcomes.

Geographical Location and Food Desert Prevalence

Geographical location plays a significant role in the prevalence of food deserts, particularly in rural and urban areas.

Urban Areas: Urban food deserts are often characterized by a lack of grocery stores and supermarkets in low-income neighborhoods. The distance between residential areas and the nearest grocery store may be substantial, requiring greater transportation efforts or reliance on convenience stores that offer limited healthy food options.

Rural Areas: Rural food deserts face unique challenges due to lower population density, limited infrastructure, and long distances from grocery stores. The absence of public transportation and the high cost of private transportation can significantly hinder residents' access to nutritious food.

Example: The Navajo Nation in the southwestern United States is an example of a rural food desert. The vast size of the reservation, combined with limited economic opportunities and geographic isolation, creates significant barriers to accessing fresh and healthy food.

Conclusion

Demographic factors such as income disparities, racial and ethnic disparities, age distribution, gender disparities, and geographical location contribute to the prevalence of food deserts. Understanding these factors is crucial in developing targeted interventions and policies to address the problem effectively.

By addressing the unique challenges faced by different demographic groups, we can work towards creating equitable access to healthy food and improving nutrition outcomes for all communities. It is essential to consider the intersectionality of these factors and implement comprehensive strategies that account for the diverse needs and experiences of individuals in food deserts. Only through a holistic and inclusive approach can we effectively combat the issue of food deserts and promote food justice for all.

International Perspective on Food Deserts

Food Desert Trends Globally

Food deserts, characterized by limited access to affordable and nutritious food, are not just a problem within the United States. They are a global issue that affects numerous countries around the world. In this section, we will explore the trends and patterns of food deserts on a global scale, understanding the common challenges and implications they pose.

Magnitude and Distribution

The prevalence of food deserts varies across countries, but the underlying factors contributing to their existence remain similar. Developing countries, in particular, face significant challenges in ensuring food security and access to nutritious food for their populations. Rapid urbanization, population growth, and inadequate infrastructure aggravate the problem, leading to the emergence of food deserts in both urban and rural areas.

In low-income countries, food deserts are often more prevalent in rural regions due to limited transportation infrastructure and lack of market integration. Insufficient access to markets, coupled with limited agricultural productivity and resources, contribute to the formation of food deserts in these areas. In urban settings, food deserts arise in areas with high poverty rates, low-income neighborhoods, and inadequate supermarket penetration.

In high-income countries, food deserts are predominantly observed in marginalized communities and areas with lower socio-economic status. Developed countries face their own set of challenges, including social inequalities, urban planning decisions, and the impact of globalization on local food systems. Despite higher overall food availability, disparities exist in terms of access to nutritious food, with disadvantaged populations bearing the brunt of this issue.

Case Studies

To gain a deeper understanding of food desert trends globally, let's explore a few case studies from different regions.

United Kingdom The United Kingdom (UK) has been a key player in addressing food deserts, with an established definition and comprehensive policy framework to combat this problem. In the UK, food deserts are more prevalent in deprived urban areas, characterized by low-income populations and limited access to supermarkets or grocery stores. The closure of local shops further exacerbates the issue.

The government and non-profit organizations have implemented various strategies to tackle food deserts in the UK. For instance, the Healthy Start program provides financial support and vouchers for pregnant women and families with young children to purchase healthy food. Additionally, initiatives like the Big Lottery Fund have invested in community-led projects to establish social supermarkets and promote local food enterprises. These efforts have had some success in reducing food insecurity and improving access to nutritious food in deprived areas.

South Africa In South Africa, food deserts are a result of a complex interplay of socio-economic disparities, historical injustices, and spatial inequalities. Apartheid-era policies and urban planning decisions have contributed to the formation of townships and informal settlements where food access is limited. These areas often lack supermarkets or formal food retail outlets, forcing residents to rely on small, unaffordable, and less nutritious corner stores or informal markets.

To combat food deserts, South Africa has implemented various government-led initiatives. One such initiative is the National School Nutrition Program, which provides free meals to millions of school children in disadvantaged areas. The program not only addresses food insecurity but also improves educational outcomes. In addition, non-profit organizations have established community gardens and food cooperatives to promote local food production and improve food access.

Australia In Australia, food deserts are predominantly observed in remote and Indigenous communities. Factors such as long distances to supermarkets, limited transport options, and high food prices contribute to food insecurity in these areas. Indigenous communities, in particular, face the dual challenge of food deserts and the loss of traditional food sources due to factors like land dispossession.

To address the issue, community-based initiatives in Australia have been playing a crucial role. For example, the Outback Stores program provides essential food items at affordable prices in remote Indigenous communities. This not only improves food access but also supports local economic development. Additionally, there are efforts to promote traditional bush foods and enhance their availability in disadvantaged areas.

Challenges and Opportunities

Food desert trends globally highlight several challenges and opportunities for addressing this complex issue.

One significant challenge is the need for infrastructure development. Access to adequate transportation systems, including roads, public transport, and delivery networks, is crucial for overcoming the spatial barriers of food deserts. Moreover, there is a need for targeted investments in supermarkets, grocery stores, and fresh food markets in underserved areas.

Another challenge is the affordability of nutritious food. In many food deserts, even when healthy food options are available, they are often more expensive than unhealthy alternatives. Ensuring that nutritious food is affordable and competitive with processed and unhealthy options is key to promoting healthier eating habits.

Opportunities lie in fostering community engagement and empowerment. Community-led initiatives, such as urban farming, community gardens, and food cooperatives, have shown promise in addressing food deserts globally. By involving local residents in the planning and implementation of solutions, these initiatives create a sense of ownership and sustainability.

Furthermore, technology can play a crucial role in bridging the gap in food access. For instance, mobile applications can provide information on nearby food sources, nutritional content, and food prices, helping individuals make informed decisions. Online platforms and food delivery services can also improve access to nutritious food, particularly in areas with limited physical retail options.

Conclusion

Food deserts are not confined to the borders of the United States; they are a global phenomenon affecting various countries and communities. Understanding the trends and challenges of food deserts globally helps us identify common issues and learn from successful interventions implemented in different regions.

By recognizing the magnitude and distribution of food deserts on a global scale, we can work towards creating effective strategies to improve food access and promote nutrition for all. Addressing food desert trends globally requires a multi-faceted approach involving government policies, community engagement, technological advancements, and a commitment to social justice and equity. It is only through collective efforts and continued research that we can strive towards a world without food deserts, ensuring that everyone has access to affordable and healthy food choices.

Case Studies of Food Deserts in Different Countries

In order to gain a comprehensive understanding of food deserts, it is important to consider case studies from different countries across the globe. While food desert trends and challenges may vary from one country to another, studying these case studies provides valuable insights into the underlying causes and potential solutions for addressing this issue. This section will explore three case studies from different countries: the United States, the United Kingdom, and Australia.

United States: South Los Angeles

One of the most well-known and extensively studied food deserts in the United States is located in South Los Angeles. This case study highlights the intersectionality of various socio-economic factors contributing to food deserts.

South Los Angeles is predominantly inhabited by low-income communities of color. Historically, the area has experienced disinvestment, racial segregation, and limited access to healthy food options. The closure of grocery stores and the prevalence of fast food chains have resulted in a lack of affordable and nutritious food choices for residents.

Studies have shown that the limited availability of fresh fruits, vegetables, and whole grains in South Los Angeles has led to higher rates of diet-related diseases, such as obesity and diabetes, among its residents. Furthermore, the lack of access to healthy food options adversely affects children's academic performance and increases the risk of developmental issues.

To address this issue, various interventions have been implemented. Initiatives like the California FreshWorks Fund have provided financing and incentives to attract supermarkets and farmers' markets to underserved areas. Additionally, community gardens, urban farming, and mobile markets have been established to increase access to fresh produce.

United Kingdom: Tower Hamlets, London

In the United Kingdom, Tower Hamlets in London serves as a compelling case study of a food desert. With a diverse population and significant income inequality, this borough faces unique challenges in terms of food access.

Tower Hamlets has a high proportion of low-income households and a significant number of residents dependent on food assistance programs. Limited availability of affordable, nutritious food options within the borough has led to poor diets and increased health inequalities.

Several interventions have aimed to alleviate the food desert conditions in Tower Hamlets. The establishment of community food hubs, such as Bow Food Bank, has provided emergency food aid and promoted healthier eating habits through cooking classes and nutrition education. Additionally, initiatives like the Tower Hamlets Food Growing Network have encouraged the creation of community gardens and allotments to increase access to fresh produce.

However, challenges persist in addressing food deserts in Tower Hamlets. Issues related to gentrification, affordability of healthy food, and long-term sustainability of interventions need to be considered for effective and equitable solutions.

Australia: Northern Territory Aboriginal Communities

In Australia, the remote Aboriginal communities in the Northern Territory present a unique case study of food deserts within an indigenous context. These communities face multiple challenges related to geography, limited infrastructure, and cultural factors.

The remote Aboriginal communities often suffer from inadequate access to fresh and nutritious food due to their isolation and the high costs associated with transporting food to these regions. Limited economic opportunities and educational resources exacerbate the issue, leading to poor health outcomes such as higher rates of malnutrition and chronic diseases.

To address food deserts in these communities, various initiatives have been implemented. The Australian government, in collaboration with indigenous organizations, has focused on improving infrastructure to enhance access to healthy food. Community-driven programs such as bush tucker initiatives, which promote traditional food sources, have also played a significant role in addressing food security and cultural preservation.

However, effective interventions require culturally appropriate approaches that respect indigenous knowledge and practices. Collaborative efforts with the community members and sustainable solutions that empower local economies are critical in ensuring long-term success.

Conclusion

Examining case studies of food deserts in different countries provides valuable insights into the complex nature of this issue and the need for context-specific solutions. The case studies presented here illustrate the importance of addressing socio-economic factors, community empowerment, and sustainability in interventions aimed at combating food deserts. By learning from successful initiatives and understanding the challenges faced in various regions, we can work towards equitable access to healthy food for all communities.

Cross-cultural comparisons and lessons learned

Understanding food deserts requires looking beyond the borders of a single country and examining the issue from a global perspective. Cross-cultural comparisons allow us to identify common challenges and effective strategies that have been implemented in different contexts. By studying food deserts in various countries, we can gain valuable insights and lessons that can inform our efforts to address this issue.

Food desert trends globally

Food deserts exist in varying degrees around the world, although they may be referred to by different names in different countries. By comparing the prevalence and characteristics of food deserts across nations, we can identify patterns and trends that shed light on the underlying causes and potential solutions.

In the United Kingdom, for example, the concept of food deserts gained significant attention in the early 2000s. Studies have shown that certain neighborhoods in the UK face similar challenges as their counterparts in the United States, with limited access to affordable and nutritious food options. The identification of food deserts in the UK prompted the development of targeted interventions and policies to address the issue.

In Canada, remote Indigenous communities often experience food insecurity and lack access to fresh produce due to their geographical isolation. This highlights the unique challenges faced by marginalized populations in food deserts and the need for culturally appropriate solutions.

In Australia, food deserts are commonly found in low-income areas and Aboriginal communities. The distance to the nearest supermarket and the high cost of healthy food are key factors contributing to food insecurity. The Australian experience emphasizes the importance of considering socioeconomic factors and the specific needs of vulnerable populations when designing interventions.

Case studies of food deserts in different countries

Examining specific case studies of food deserts in different countries allows us to delve deeper into the unique cultural, geographical, and economic factors that shape the problem and potential solutions. Here are a few examples:

1. Japan: Despite being a highly developed country with a robust food system, Japan faces challenges in rural areas where large supermarket chains are often concentrated in urban centers. This has led to the emergence of food deserts in rural communities, primarily affecting older adults and low-income individuals. The Japanese government has implemented initiatives to support local agriculture and improve access to fresh produce in these areas.

2. South Africa: Urban townships in South Africa face food deserts due to a combination of historical inequalities, rapid urbanization, and limited economic opportunities. These areas often lack supermarkets and have an overreliance on small, informal food outlets with limited healthy options. Community-based initiatives, such as urban farming and cooperative grocery stores, have been successful in addressing food insecurity and revitalizing local economies.

3. Brazil: In Brazil, urban slums known as favelas are characterized by limited access to nutritious food and high rates of poverty. Non-profit organizations and grassroots movements have implemented innovative solutions, such as community kitchens and mobile food markets, to alleviate food insecurity in these vulnerable communities.

Cross-cultural lessons learned

Cross-cultural comparisons offer valuable lessons for addressing food deserts and promoting food justice globally. Here are some key lessons learned:

1. Context matters: Solutions for food deserts must be tailored to the specific cultural, economic, and geographic context of each region. A one-size-fits-all approach is unlikely to be successful.

2. Collaborative approaches: Engaging local communities, non-profit organizations, government agencies, and private sector stakeholders is crucial for developing comprehensive and sustainable interventions. Collaborative approaches ensure that diverse perspectives are represented and that solutions are built on shared knowledge and experiences.

3. Policy support: Strong government policies and initiatives play a critical role in addressing food deserts. Legislation that supports the establishment of grocery stores in underserved areas, incentivizes local agriculture, and promotes healthy food options is essential.

4. Empowerment and education: Empowering individuals with knowledge about nutrition, food preparation, and gardening can foster self-reliance and resilience in food deserts. Education campaigns and community workshops can have a lasting impact on improving dietary choices and food access.

5. Multi-sectoral approaches: Solving the problem of food deserts requires collaboration across sectors, including health, education, transportation, and urban planning. By integrating efforts and resources, it is possible to create a comprehensive and sustainable framework for addressing food deserts.

Resources for further exploration

For further exploration of cross-cultural comparisons and lessons learned in the context of food deserts, the following resources are recommended:

1. "Food Justice" by Robert Gottlieb and Anupama Joshi: This book provides a comprehensive analysis of food justice issues, including cross-cultural perspectives and case studies from different countries.

2. The Food and Agriculture Organization (FAO) of the United Nations: The FAO website offers a wealth of information and publications on food security and access, including case studies and best practices from around the world.

3. "Food Deserts and Health Inequities" by Ronald Stolk and Marloes Trienekens: This research article explores cross-national differences in food deserts and their impact on health, providing valuable insights into the global dimension of the issue.

Exercises

1. Research and identify a country or region that has successfully implemented policies or interventions to address food deserts. Describe the strategies that were employed and evaluate their effectiveness in improving food access and nutrition outcomes.

2. In your community or neighborhood, identify a potential food desert and propose a multi-sectoral approach to address the issue. Consider factors such as transportation, education, and policy changes in your intervention plan.

3. Investigate a cultural practice or traditional food system that promotes food security and access in a specific community or country. Discuss how this practice can be leveraged to address food deserts in other contexts.

4. Interview someone from a marginalized community who has experienced food insecurity or limited food access. Use their insights and personal experiences to identify key challenges and potential solutions for addressing food deserts in their community.

Remember, food deserts are complex issues rooted in socioeconomic disparities and structural inequalities. It is crucial to approach these exercises with sensitivity, respect, and the understanding that solutions require holistic and inclusive approaches.

Theoretical Frameworks for Understanding Food Deserts

Socioeconomic Theories

Socioeconomic theories play a crucial role in understanding the complex dynamics of food deserts. These theories examine the relationship between societal factors, economic conditions, and the distribution of resources within a community. By exploring the socioeconomic dimensions of food deserts, we can gain insights into the underlying causes and potential solutions for this issue.

Neoclassical Economics

Neoclassical economics is a fundamental theory that provides insights into the functioning of markets and the allocation of resources. According to neoclassical economics, individuals act rationally to maximize their utility, and markets efficiently allocate resources based on supply and demand. However, this theory fails to explain the persistence of food deserts in low-income communities.

In the context of food deserts, neoclassical economics suggests that the absence of grocery stores in these areas is due to low demand. It argues that residents in food deserts may have lower purchasing power, limited preferences for healthy foods, or face transportation barriers. As a result, businesses are reluctant to invest in these areas, leading to limited access to affordable and nutritious food options.

Social Stratification Theory

Social stratification theory examines the unequal distribution of resources, privileges, and opportunities in society. It highlights the role of social class, income, and education as determinants of access to various goods, including food. In the context of food deserts, social stratification theory suggests that individuals from lower socioeconomic backgrounds are more likely to reside in these areas.

According to this theory, individuals with higher socioeconomic status have better access to quality foods due to their greater purchasing power and education. They can afford to live in neighborhoods with supermarkets and have the means to travel to other areas to access a variety of food options. In contrast, individuals with lower socioeconomic status may be constrained by limited income, educational opportunities, and transportation options, making them more susceptible to living in food deserts.

Food Justice Framework

The food justice framework encompasses a broader perspective on food deserts by examining the structural causes and systemic inequalities that contribute to this issue. It acknowledges the intersections of race, class, and socioeconomics, emphasizing the importance of social and economic justice in addressing food access disparities.

According to the food justice framework, food deserts are not a natural outcome of market forces or individual choices but are a manifestation of systemic injustices. It highlights the historical and ongoing factors, such as redlining, discriminatory lending practices, and zoning policies, that have shaped the geography of food deserts. This perspective calls for a comprehensive approach that addresses socioeconomic disparities, promotes community empowerment, and advocates for policy changes to ensure equitable access to healthy and affordable food for all individuals.

Sustainable Development Goals

The United Nations' Sustainable Development Goals (SDGs) provide a global framework for addressing poverty, hunger, and inequality. SDG 2 aims to end hunger, achieve food security, improve nutrition, and promote sustainable agriculture. In the context of food deserts, the SDGs emphasize the need for targeted interventions and policies that address the root causes of food disparities.

The SDGs recognize the interconnectedness of various factors contributing to food deserts, such as poverty, education, health, and urban planning. By adopting a multidimensional approach, the SDGs emphasize the importance of collaborative efforts and cross-sectoral partnerships to promote inclusive and sustainable food systems. This framework encourages the alignment of economic, social, and environmental goals to tackle the complex issue of food deserts.

Example: The Impact of Gentrification

Gentrification is a socioeconomic process characterized by the influx of higher-income residents into low-income neighborhoods, often resulting in rising property values and the displacement of existing residents. While gentrification can bring economic development and amenities to previously neglected areas, it can also exacerbate food access disparities, leading to the emergence of new food deserts.

For example, let's consider a low-income neighborhood that undergoes gentrification. As property values rise, existing residents may be unable to afford the higher rents or property taxes, forcing them to relocate to areas with limited access to affordable groceries. As a result, the gentrified neighborhood may attract new businesses that cater to the tastes and preferences of the incoming affluent residents, potentially leaving behind the remaining lower-income residents with even fewer food options.

To address the socioeconomic impact of gentrification on food access, policymakers and urban planners need to consider strategies that prioritize community engagement, affordable housing, and the retention of existing local businesses. This example illustrates the need to address socioeconomic factors comprehensively to prevent the displacement of vulnerable populations and the emergence of new food deserts.

Conclusion

Socioeconomic theories provide valuable insights into the complex dynamics of food deserts and their impact on nutrition and health. Neoclassical economics, social stratification theory, the food justice framework, and the Sustainable Development Goals offer different perspectives on the causes and potential solutions for food deserts. By adopting a multidimensional approach that addresses systemic barriers to access and promotes equitable food systems, we can work towards creating sustainable and healthy communities for all.

Health Disparities and Food Access

Access to healthy and nutritious food is a crucial determinant of health. However, in food deserts, where there is limited availability of affordable and quality food options, individuals often face significant barriers to accessing nutritious food. This section explores the relationship between health disparities and food access, highlighting the impact of food deserts on population health and well-being.

Nutrition-related Health Disparities

Health disparities refer to differences in health outcomes and access to healthcare services between different population groups. Nutrition-related health disparities are particularly evident in food deserts, as individuals residing in these areas have limited access to fresh fruits, vegetables, whole grains, and other essential food items. As a result, they are more likely to consume a diet that is high in processed foods, unhealthy fats, and added sugars.

The lack of access to nutritious food options in food deserts contributes to various health disparities, including:

- **Obesity:** Individuals living in food deserts are at a higher risk of obesity due to the limited availability of healthy food choices. The consumption of energy-dense, nutrient-poor foods in these areas contributes to excessive calorie intake and weight gain.

- **Cardiovascular diseases:** The consumption of a diet high in saturated fats and added sugars, commonly found in processed foods, increases the risk of cardiovascular diseases such as hypertension, heart disease, and stroke.

- **Type 2 diabetes:** The lack of access to fresh fruits and vegetables, whole grains, and lean proteins, coupled with the consumption of high-calorie processed foods, is associated with an increased risk of developing type 2 diabetes.

- **Micronutrient deficiencies:** Limited access to fresh produce and nutrient-rich foods increases the risk of micronutrient deficiencies, leading to impaired immune function, poor growth and development, and a higher susceptibility to infections.

Food Access and Chronic Diseases

Food access plays a pivotal role in the development and management of chronic diseases. Individuals living in food deserts face challenges in maintaining a healthy diet, which can have long-term implications for their health. The lack of access to nutritious food options contributes to the development and exacerbation of chronic diseases, such as:

- **Hypertension:** The consumption of a diet high in sodium, commonly found in processed foods, coupled with the limited availability of fresh fruits and vegetables, contributes to the development of hypertension.
- **Coronary artery disease:** The consumption of a diet high in trans fats and added sugars, commonly found in processed foods, increases the risk of developing coronary artery disease.
- **Cancer:** Limited access to fresh fruits, vegetables, and whole grains, which are rich in antioxidants and phytochemicals, is associated with an increased risk of certain types of cancer, such as colorectal and breast cancer.

The impact of food deserts on chronic disease outcomes is further exacerbated by socioeconomic factors, such as limited financial resources and educational attainment, which can influence individuals' ability to make healthier food choices.

Addressing Health Disparities in Food Deserts

Reducing health disparities related to food access requires a multifaceted approach that addresses various determinants of health. Some strategies to improve food access and reduce health disparities in food deserts include:

- **Expansion of healthy food retail:** Increasing the availability of affordable and nutritious food options in food deserts through the establishment of supermarkets, grocery stores, and farmers markets.
- **Mobile food markets:** Implementing mobile food markets that bring fresh produce and healthy food options directly to underserved communities, increasing accessibility for individuals without reliable transportation.

- **Community gardens and urban farming:** Promoting community gardens and urban farming initiatives to empower communities to grow their own produce and increase access to fresh fruits and vegetables.
- **Nutrition education:** Providing nutrition education programs and resources to empower individuals with knowledge and skills to make healthier choices within the constraints of their food environment.
- **Policy changes:** Advocating for policy changes at the local, state, and federal levels to address structural inequities and support initiatives aimed at improving access to healthy food in food deserts.

It is important to recognize that addressing health disparities in food deserts requires a comprehensive and collaborative effort involving various stakeholders, including policymakers, community organizations, healthcare providers, and individuals themselves. By implementing these strategies and promoting equitable access to nutritious food, we can work towards reducing health disparities and improving the overall health and well-being of populations residing in food deserts.

Environmental justice and food deserts

Environmental justice is a concept that recognizes the unequal distribution of environmental burdens and benefits among different populations, particularly marginalized communities. It focuses on the intersection of social and environmental issues, and aims to address the disproportionate impacts of environmental hazards on vulnerable populations.

When examining the issue of food deserts through an environmental justice lens, it becomes clear that there is a connection between the lack of access to healthy food and the structural inequalities that certain communities face. Environmental injustice manifests in the form of limited access to fresh and nutritious food, often resulting from discriminatory practices and policies that perpetuate socioeconomic disparities.

1. Historical context of environmental justice: The history of environmental justice can be traced back to the civil rights movement in the United States during the 1960s and 1970s. Activists started raising awareness about how marginalized communities, particularly communities of color, were disproportionately burdened by environmental hazards such as pollution and toxic waste sites. Over time, the environmental justice movement gained momentum and began to address other aspects of environmental inequality, including food access.

2. Structural factors contributing to food deserts: The emergence of food deserts can be linked to a range of structural factors, many of which have roots in systemic racism and economic disparities. These factors include:

a) Residential segregation: Racial and socioeconomic segregation have played a significant role in the creation and persistence of food deserts. Low-income communities and communities of color are often concentrated in areas with limited access to supermarkets and grocery stores that offer fresh, affordable, and healthy food options.

b) Redlining and disinvestment: Historical discriminatory practices like redlining, which involved the denial of housing loans to certain neighborhoods based on race, have led to disinvestment in predominantly minority communities. These areas often lack the infrastructure and resources necessary for the establishment of grocery stores and fresh food retailers.

c) Land use and zoning policies: Land use and zoning policies can perpetuate inequities in food access by limiting or restricting the establishment of supermarkets and grocery stores in low-income areas. This can result in a lack of healthy food options and an overabundance of fast food restaurants and convenience stores that predominantly offer processed and unhealthy foods.

3. Environmental justice implications of food deserts: Food deserts intersect with environmental justice issues in several ways:

a) Health disparities: The lack of access to healthy food options in food deserts contributes to higher rates of diet-related health problems, such as obesity, diabetes, and heart disease, among marginalized communities. This perpetuates health disparities and exacerbates existing inequities in health outcomes.

b) Environmental pollution: Food deserts are often located in areas with higher levels of environmental pollution, such as industrial zones or neighborhoods close to highways. The increased exposure to environmental toxins and pollutants further compromises the health and well-being of residents in these communities.

c) Displacement and gentrification: As efforts are made to address food deserts, there is a risk of unintended consequences, such as displacement and gentrification. When supermarkets or other food retailers enter low-income communities to fill the food access gap, it can lead to increased property values and the subsequent displacement of existing residents. This raises important questions about the social and economic impacts of food justice initiatives.

4. Strategies for addressing environmental justice in food deserts: In order to promote environmental justice in the context of food deserts, it is crucial to address the root causes of inequality and engage in comprehensive and inclusive interventions. Some strategies include:

a) Community engagement and empowerment: Engaging affected communities in the decision-making processes is essential for ensuring that their voices are heard and that interventions are tailored to their specific needs. Building partnerships with community organizations and involving residents in initiatives such as community gardens and farmers markets can empower communities to take control of their food systems.

b) Policy and advocacy: Advocacy for policy changes at the local, state, and federal levels is necessary to address the systemic issues that contribute to food deserts. This can involve advocating for zoning changes, incentives for grocery store development in underserved areas, and increased funding for nutrition programs.

c) Sustainable and equitable food systems: Building sustainable food systems that prioritize local food production, reduce environmental impacts, and ensure equitable access to fresh and nutritious food is a key component of addressing environmental justice in food deserts. This can include supporting urban agriculture initiatives, expanding farmers markets, and promoting alternative food distribution models that prioritize community needs.

d) Education and awareness: Providing nutrition education and promoting awareness about the importance of healthy eating can empower individuals to make informed food choices. This can be done through educational programs in schools, community centers, and healthcare facilities.

In order to create long-lasting change, it is important to acknowledge and address the systemic issues that underlie food deserts. By incorporating the principles of environmental justice into interventions, we can work towards creating healthier and more equitable food systems for all communities.

Socioeconomic Factors and Food Deserts

Poverty and Economic Inequality

Poverty Rates and Food Access

Poverty is a critical factor that contributes to the existence of food deserts. In this section, we will explore the relationship between poverty rates and food access, examining how low-income communities face significant challenges in accessing healthy and affordable food options.

Understanding Poverty Rates

Poverty is a multidimensional concept that encompasses both income and living conditions. It is typically defined by an individual or household's inability to meet basic needs, such as food, shelter, and clothing. Poverty rates are often measured as the percentage of the population living below the poverty line, which is determined by the government based on income thresholds.

The poverty line varies across countries and regions, taking into account the cost of living and local economic conditions. In the United States, for instance, the poverty line is defined by the Department of Health and Human Services based on annual income levels.

Poverty rates are crucial indicators of socioeconomic well-being and are used to assess the extent of poverty within a population. These rates provide insights into the income disparities and economic inequalities that exist within a society.

Impact of Poverty on Food Access

Poverty has a significant impact on food access, particularly in low-income communities. As individuals and families struggle to meet their basic needs, accessing healthy and affordable food becomes a daily challenge. Several key factors contribute to the limited food access faced by individuals living in poverty:

1. Limited financial resources: Poverty often means having a restricted budget for food expenditures. This limitation makes it difficult for individuals to afford nutritious food options, such as fresh fruits, vegetables, and lean meats, which tend to be more expensive than processed and unhealthy alternatives.

2. Limited proximity to grocery stores: Low-income neighborhoods and rural areas are often characterized by a lack of nearby grocery stores. This limited proximity creates a barrier to accessing fresh and healthy food options. Instead, residents may rely on convenience stores and fast food outlets that offer predominantly processed and unhealthy food choices.

3. Transportation barriers: Many low-income individuals do not have access to private vehicles, relying instead on public transportation or walking. This reliance on public transportation can limit their ability to travel long distances to reach grocery stores with affordable and nutritious food options. As a result, they may be forced to rely on local corner stores or convenience stores, where the variety of fresh and healthy foods is limited.

4. Food affordability: In areas with limited food options, the cost of food can be disproportionately higher due to reduced competition among retailers. This high cost of food in food deserts further exacerbates the challenges faced by low-income individuals, making it even more difficult to afford nutritious options.

5. Lack of food assistance programs: Although government assistance programs like the Supplemental Nutrition Assistance Program (SNAP) exist to support individuals living in poverty, their reach and impact are often limited. Some individuals may not be aware of such programs or may face challenges in accessing and utilizing them effectively.

The combination of these factors leads to a situation where individuals living in poverty often experience limited food options that are high in calories, saturated fats, and added sugars but low in essential nutrients. This can contribute to poor dietary habits and negative health outcomes, such as obesity, diabetes, and cardiovascular diseases.

Addressing Poverty and Food Access

Addressing poverty is a crucial step in improving food access and reducing the prevalence of food deserts. It requires a comprehensive approach that combines social policies, economic interventions, and community-based initiatives. Here are some potential strategies for addressing poverty and improving food access:

1. Employment and income support: Creating employment opportunities and promoting stable income sources can help individuals and families lift themselves out of poverty. Providing job training programs, increasing the minimum wage, and expanding income support programs are important steps in addressing poverty and its impact on food access.

2. Affordable housing initiatives: Access to affordable and safe housing is essential in addressing poverty. Stable housing can free up financial resources for individuals to allocate towards basic needs, such as food. Implementing affordable housing initiatives can improve the overall well-being of low-income communities and enhance their access to healthy food options.

3. Community economic development: Encouraging the development of local businesses and cooperatives in low-income communities can help address food access issues. Cultivating an environment that supports entrepreneurship and local economic growth can lead to the establishment of grocery stores, farmers markets, and community gardens that offer affordable and nutritious food choices.

4. Collaboration and advocacy: Building partnerships between community organizations, local businesses, and government agencies is crucial in addressing the systemic issues that contribute to poverty and food deserts. Engaging in advocacy efforts and influencing policy changes can create a more supportive environment for low-income communities, improving their access to healthy and affordable food options.

By focusing on poverty reduction and promoting economic opportunities, communities can create an environment that supports food security and access to nutritious food options. It is crucial to address the root causes of poverty and collaborate across sectors to ensure sustainable solutions that benefit all individuals, regardless of their socioeconomic status.

In the next section, we will explore the role of transportation in food access, highlighting the challenges faced by individuals living in food deserts and the potential solutions to improve their mobility and reach to nutritious food options.

Income Disparities and Healthy Food Options

Income is a significant determinant of food access and choices in food deserts. Low-income individuals and families often face economic constraints that limit their ability to afford and access healthy food options. This section explores the relationship between income disparities and healthy food options, examining the impact of income on food insecurity and the strategies employed to address this issue.

The Link Between Poverty and Food Access

Poverty rates have a direct correlation with food access and availability in food deserts. Low-income communities tend to have limited resources and face challenges in accessing nutritious foods. As a result, these communities often rely on cheap and unhealthy food options, such as fast food and processed foods, which are readily available but lack nutritional value.

Furthermore, income disparities contribute to unequal distribution of supermarkets and grocery stores. Affluent neighborhoods typically have better access to full-service grocery stores with a wide variety of fresh and healthy food options. On the other hand, low-income neighborhoods are often characterized by a lack of supermarkets, leaving residents with limited choices and relying on convenience stores or small corner stores that offer unhealthy and overpriced food items.

Income Inequality and Healthy Food Pricing

One of the key issues in food deserts is the high cost of healthy food options compared to unhealthy alternatives. Low-income individuals and families often struggle to afford fresh fruits, vegetables, and whole grains due to the higher prices associated with these items. On the other hand, highly processed and unhealthy foods, such as sugary drinks and snacks, tend to be more affordable and readily available.

The concept of a "healthy food premium" refers to the additional cost of purchasing nutritious food items. This premium is often attributed to various factors, including production and distribution costs, as well as the economies of scale enjoyed by manufacturers of unhealthy processed foods. As a result, low-income individuals are more likely to experience the trade-off between limited financial resources and healthy food choices, often compromising their nutrition due to financial constraints.

Solutions for Addressing Income Disparities and Healthy Food Options

Addressing income disparities and their impact on healthy food options requires multi-faceted approaches that target both the supply and demand sides of the problem. The following strategies have been employed to improve access to affordable and nutritious food in low-income communities:

1. **Increased funding for food assistance programs:** Government-led initiatives, such as the Supplemental Nutrition Assistance Program (SNAP), aim to provide low-income individuals with financial assistance to purchase nutritious food.

2. **Improving income and employment opportunities:** Efforts to reduce income disparities and increase employment opportunities in low-income communities can help individuals and families afford healthier food options.

3. **Promoting community gardens and urban farming:** Community gardens and urban farming initiatives empower individuals to grow their own fruits, vegetables, and herbs, thereby increasing access to fresh and affordable produce.

4. **Establishing farmers markets and cooperatives:** Farmers markets and food cooperatives can provide direct access to fresh and locally sourced produce at lower prices, thereby addressing the healthy food premium in low-income neighborhoods.

5. **Collaborative efforts with food retailers:** Engaging with food retailers, including large supermarket chains, to open stores in food deserts can promote the availability of affordable and healthy food options.

6. **Supporting local food enterprises:** Encouraging the establishment of local food enterprises, such as community-supported agriculture (CSA) programs and mobile markets, can increase access to fresh and nutritious food in underserved areas.

It is important to note that successful interventions should be tailored to the specific needs and characteristics of each community. A comprehensive approach that combines policies, economic development, and community engagement is essential for addressing income disparities and ensuring access to healthy food options in food deserts.

Case Study: The Healthy Neighborhoods Program

One example of a program that addresses income disparities and healthy food options is the Healthy Neighborhoods Program in Baltimore, Maryland. The program aims to increase access to healthy food in low-income neighborhoods by supporting the establishment and expansion of grocery stores and improving the availability of fresh and affordable produce.

In collaboration with local government agencies, community organizations, and private investors, the program provides financing and technical assistance to grocery store operators and developers interested in opening or expanding stores in underserved areas. This includes offering low-interest loans, grants for physical improvements, and sales support programs.

The Healthy Neighborhoods Program also includes initiatives to increase nutrition education and promote healthy food choices among residents. These efforts involve partnering with local organizations to offer nutrition workshops, cooking demonstrations, and other educational activities, helping individuals make informed decisions and adopt healthier eating habits.

Preliminary evaluations of the program have shown promising results, including increased access to healthy food options in underserved neighborhoods, improved availability of fresh produce, and increased community engagement. The Healthy Neighborhoods Program serves as an example of a comprehensive approach that addresses income disparities while promoting healthier food options for low-income communities.

Conclusion

Income disparities play a significant role in shaping the food options available to individuals and families in food deserts. Limited financial resources and the higher cost of healthy food options contribute to the prevalence of unhealthy diets and food insecurity in low-income communities. Addressing these disparities requires a multi-faceted approach, including policy changes, economic development, and community-based initiatives.

By implementing strategies that increase access to affordable and nutritious food, such as supporting local food enterprises, promoting community gardens, and collaborating with food retailers, it is possible to mitigate the impact of income disparities on healthy food options. These efforts, in combination with nutrition education and community engagement, can contribute to building healthier and more equitable food environments in food deserts.

Exercises

1. Research a local food assistance program in your community. What are the eligibility criteria? How does it contribute to improving access to healthy food options for low-income individuals and families?

2. Visit a nearby farmers market or food cooperative and compare the prices of fresh produce to those at a local convenience store. Analyze the cost difference and discuss how these disparities can impact the food choices of low-income individuals.

3. Identify an innovative solution or intervention that has been implemented in a food desert to address income disparities and improve healthy food options. Assess its effectiveness and discuss any challenges or limitations it may face.

4. Conduct a survey or interview individuals in a low-income neighborhood to understand their perception of the availability and affordability of healthy food options. Analyze the feedback and propose potential strategies to address the identified barriers.

Additional Resources

1. Cummins, S., Flint, E., & Matthews, S. A. (2014). New neighborhood grocery store increased awareness of food access but did not alter dietary habits or obesity. Health Affairs, 33(2), 283-291.

2. Gittelsohn, J., Rowan, M., & Gadhoke, P. (2012). Interventions in small food stores to change the food environment, improve diet, and reduce risk of chronic disease. Preventing Chronic Disease, 9, E59.

3. Walker, R. E., Keane, C. R., & Burke, J. G. (2010). Disparities and access to healthy food in the United States: A review of food deserts literature. Health & Place, 16(5), 876-884.

4. Wrigley, N., Warm, D., & Margetts, B. (2003). Deprivation, diet, and food-retail access: Finding from the Leeds 'food deserts' study. Environment and Planning A, 35(1), 151-188.

Socioeconomic patterns and food deserts

Socioeconomic factors play a significant role in the emergence and persistence of food deserts. In this section, we will explore the relationship between poverty, income disparities, and food access. We will also examine the impact of socioeconomic patterns on the prevalence and severity of food deserts in different communities.

Poverty rates and food access

Poverty is a major socioeconomic factor that contributes to the existence of food deserts. When individuals and households lack the financial resources to meet their basic needs, including accessing nutritious food, they are more likely to live in areas with limited food options. High poverty rates are often accompanied by a lack of nearby grocery stores or supermarkets that provide a variety of fresh and healthy food choices.

Research has consistently shown a strong correlation between poverty rates and the presence of food deserts. For example, a study conducted in urban areas of the United States found that neighborhoods with higher poverty rates were more likely to have limited access to supermarkets and higher concentrations of fast food restaurants. This pattern demonstrates the unequal distribution of food resources and the challenges faced by low-income communities in obtaining healthy food options.

Addressing poverty is crucial to addressing food deserts. Efforts should be made to improve economic opportunities, increase affordable housing options, and provide financial assistance to individuals and families living in poverty. It is also important to advocate for policies that promote income equality and address socioeconomic disparities, as these underlying factors contribute to the creation and perpetuation of food deserts.

Income disparities and healthy food options

Income disparities also play a significant role in shaping the food landscape and availability of healthy food options. Low-income communities often have limited access to high-quality grocery stores and farmers markets that offer fresh produce and a wide range of nutritious foods. On the other hand, wealthier communities typically have greater access to these resources and can afford to purchase healthier food options.

The income disparities in food access contribute to the unequal distribution of food deserts. Individuals and families with higher incomes can afford to travel longer distances to access nutritious food, while those with lower incomes may rely on convenience stores or fast food establishments located within their neighborhoods. The lack of affordable and healthy food options in low-income areas further exacerbates existing health disparities and perpetuates the cycle of poverty.

To address income disparities in food access, it is important to increase the availability of affordable and nutritious food options in low-income communities. This can be achieved through initiatives such as subsidizing healthy food purchases, incentivizing the establishment of grocery stores and farmers markets in underserved areas, and implementing policies that promote fair wages and income equality. Additionally, efforts to improve financial literacy and budgeting skills can help individuals make informed decisions about food purchasing and prioritize healthy options within their limited budgets.

Socioeconomic patterns and food deserts

Socioeconomic patterns have a profound impact on the prevalence and severity of food deserts in different communities. Urban areas with higher poverty rates and income disparities are more likely to have concentrated food deserts, while rural areas often face unique challenges related to access due to limited transportation options and geographic isolation.

For instance, in urban food deserts, the lack of affordable and nutritious food options is often compounded by limited transportation options. Low-income individuals may rely on public transportation or walking to access grocery stores, and the availability and reliability of these transportation modes may be compromised in disadvantaged neighborhoods. This further limits their ability to access healthy food options outside their immediate vicinity.

In rural food deserts, limited access to transportation, particularly for those without personal vehicles, poses a significant challenge. The distances between grocery stores or farmers markets may be substantial, making it difficult for individuals to travel and obtain fresh and healthy food regularly. Additionally, the limited population density and market demand in rural areas may discourage businesses from establishing grocery stores, exacerbating the problem of food access.

Addressing socioeconomic patterns and their impact on food deserts requires comprehensive strategies that consider the unique challenges faced by different communities. Efforts should be focused on improving both transportation infrastructure and food retail options in urban areas, as well as developing innovative solutions to overcome transportation barriers in rural areas.

Collaborative partnerships between government agencies, community organizations, and businesses can help create sustainable solutions that address the underlying socioeconomic factors contributing to food deserts.

In conclusion, socioeconomic patterns and disparities, including poverty rates and income inequalities, significantly influence the prevalence and severity of food deserts. These factors shape the availability and accessibility of healthy food options, creating barriers for low-income individuals and communities. Addressing these underlying socioeconomic issues and implementing targeted interventions are essential for alleviating food deserts and promoting equitable access to nutritious food for all.

Access to Transportation

Transportation Barriers in Food Deserts

Transportation plays a critical role in determining access to food in food deserts. In this section, we will explore the various transportation barriers faced by individuals living in food deserts and discuss potential solutions to address these challenges.

Limited Public Transportation Options

One of the primary transportation barriers in food deserts is the lack of reliable and affordable public transportation options. Many residents in these areas do not own a car or have limited access to private transportation, making it difficult for them to travel to grocery stores or supermarkets located outside their neighborhoods. This issue is particularly prevalent in low-income urban areas where public transportation systems may be inadequate or nonexistent.

The lack of efficient public transportation creates a vicious cycle, as the absence of grocery stores in food deserts discourages investment in public transportation, and the absence of reliable public transportation makes it difficult for residents to access healthy food options outside their immediate neighborhoods.

Example: Consider a low-income neighborhood in a city where the nearest grocery store is several miles away. Residents in this community rely heavily on public transportation, but the available bus routes do not directly connect to the grocery store. As a result, individuals must take multiple buses or transfer frequently, significantly increasing their travel time and making grocery shopping a cumbersome task.

Inadequate Infrastructure

Another transportation barrier in food deserts is the lack of infrastructure to support transportation options. In many cases, grocery stores and supermarkets are located in areas with better infrastructure, such as well-maintained roads, sidewalks, and bike lanes. However, these amenities may be lacking or poorly developed in food desert neighborhoods.

The absence of proper infrastructure makes it unsafe and challenging for residents to commute to grocery stores on foot, bicycles, or other alternative modes of transportation. This lack of infrastructure restricts individuals' options to reach healthy food sources, further exacerbating the food access problem in these areas.

Example: Imagine a rural food desert community with limited options for transportation. The roads leading to the nearest grocery store are poorly maintained and lack proper pedestrian walkways or bike lanes. As a result, residents face significant safety risks while attempting to walk or cycle to the store, discouraging them from making these alternative transportation choices.

Solution: Community Transportation Initiatives

To tackle transportation barriers in food deserts, community transportation initiatives can play a vital role. These initiatives aim to provide accessible and affordable transportation options specifically tailored to the needs of residents in food deserts.

Collaborative Transportation Networks: One strategy is to establish collaborative transportation networks where community members voluntarily offer rides to others in need. This can be facilitated through online platforms or community organizations, connecting individuals who have cars with those who require transportation to grocery stores or supermarkets.

Mobile Grocery Stores: Another innovative approach is the introduction of mobile grocery stores. These are specially designed vehicles equipped with fresh produce and other grocery items that travel to different food desert neighborhoods on a scheduled basis. This initiative not only eliminates the need for transportation to distant grocery stores but also brings healthy food options directly to the community's doorstep.

Improving Infrastructure: Investing in infrastructure improvements, such as enhancing public transportation routes, creating safe pedestrian walkways, and installing bike lanes, can significantly enhance transportation options in food deserts. These improvements make it easier and safer for individuals to access grocery stores and supermarkets using alternative modes of transportation.

Advocacy for Policy Change

In addition to community-driven solutions, advocacy for policy change at the local, state, and federal levels is crucial to address transportation barriers in food deserts effectively. Government policies and initiatives can provide the necessary funding and support to develop and improve transportation infrastructure and services in these underserved areas.

Transportation Equity: Advocating for transportation equity policies can ensure that resources are allocated fairly, prioritizing investments in low-income neighborhoods and communities experiencing transportation challenges. This includes advocating for increased public transportation options, better connectivity to grocery stores, and improved infrastructure in food deserts.

Public-Private Partnerships: Encouraging public-private partnerships can also facilitate innovative transportation solutions in food deserts. Collaborations between government entities, transportation companies, and community organizations can lead to the development of innovative transportation models specifically targeted at improving food access and reducing transportation barriers.

Conclusion

Transportation barriers in food deserts pose significant challenges for individuals seeking access to healthy food options. Limited public transportation options and inadequate infrastructure hinder residents' ability to travel to grocery stores located outside their neighborhoods. Community transportation initiatives and advocacy for policy change are essential in addressing these barriers. Collaborative transportation networks, mobile grocery stores, and infrastructure improvements contribute to improving transportation options, making healthy food more accessible in food deserts. Advocacy efforts for equitable transportation policies further support long-term solutions to address transportation challenges and ensure that all individuals have equal access to healthy food choices.

Public transportation and food access

Access to transportation plays a crucial role in determining food access and overcoming the challenges posed by food deserts. Many individuals living in food deserts lack personal vehicles or have limited mobility options, making it difficult for them to travel long distances to reach grocery stores or markets that offer healthy and affordable food options. This section will explore the relationship between public transportation and food access, highlighting the impact of transport barriers on food deserts and presenting innovative solutions to address this issue.

Transportation barriers in food deserts

Transportation barriers are a significant challenge faced by individuals living in food deserts. Limited availability and accessibility of public transportation options make it challenging for residents to travel to grocery stores and other food retailers. This barrier is particularly acute for those who do not have access to a private vehicle and rely solely on public transportation.

Several factors contribute to transportation barriers in food deserts. First, there may be a lack of nearby bus stops or train stations, forcing residents to walk long distances to access public transportation. This is a significant issue for individuals with mobility limitations or those who have young children with them. Second, public transportation may have limited operating hours, making it difficult for individuals to travel to grocery stores during off-peak hours or after work.

Furthermore, the affordability of public transportation can also be a hurdle for residents of food deserts. Low-income individuals may struggle to afford the cost of bus or train fare, making it financially burdensome to rely on public transportation regularly.

Public transportation and food access

Improving public transportation systems can have significant implications for alleviating food access issues in food deserts. Better transportation options can connect residents to grocery stores and farmers markets, enabling them to access fresh and healthy food within a reasonable distance.

One approach to address transportation barriers is to enhance the coverage and frequency of public transportation routes in food deserts. This can include increasing the number of bus stops or adding new routes that specifically connect these areas to supermarkets and food retailers. Moreover, extending the operating hours of public transportation can ensure that residents have the flexibility to travel to and from grocery stores at convenient times.

Another innovative solution is the implementation of free or subsidized transportation programs for residents of food deserts. These programs can include discounted bus or train fares, transportation vouchers, or partnerships with rideshare companies to provide affordable transportation options. By reducing the financial burden of transportation, these initiatives can significantly improve accessibility to food retailers for low-income individuals.

Collaboration between public transportation agencies and community organizations is also crucial in addressing transportation challenges in food deserts. By working together, these stakeholders can identify the specific needs of the community and develop tailored transportation solutions that meet the unique requirements of residents. This collaborative approach can ensure that transportation services are responsive to the needs of individuals living in food deserts.

Innovative solutions for improving transportation in food deserts

In addition to traditional public transportation options, innovative approaches using technology can enhance transportation access in food deserts. For example, the utilization of mobile apps can help residents plan their grocery shopping trips by providing real-time information on bus schedules, routes, and estimated travel times. These apps can also offer navigation features, ensuring that individuals can reach their desired food retail locations efficiently.

Furthermore, shared mobility services, such as bike-sharing or carpooling programs, can supplement existing public transportation options in food deserts. These services can provide additional flexibility for residents, enabling them to access grocery stores that may not be directly served by public transportation routes. For example, bike-sharing programs can offer an inexpensive and environmentally friendly mode of transportation for short-distance trips to nearby grocery stores.

Engaging community members in the design and implementation of transportation solutions is crucial for their success. This can involve establishing community-led transportation advisory boards or holding public meetings to gather input and feedback from residents. By involving the community in decision-making processes, transportation initiatives can be better tailored to meet the specific needs and preferences of food desert residents.

To assess the effectiveness of transportation interventions, data collection and evaluation are essential. This can involve tracking the number of individuals using public transportation to access food retailers, surveying residents to gauge their satisfaction with transportation services, and monitoring changes in food access indicators, such as the distance residents need to travel to reach a grocery store.

In conclusion, public transportation plays a vital role in addressing food access challenges in food deserts. By improving transportation options and reducing barriers, individuals living in these areas can more easily reach grocery stores and farmers markets. Innovative solutions, such as expanding public transportation routes, implementing free or subsidized transportation programs, and leveraging technology, can help ensure equitable access to healthy and affordable food for all residents, regardless of their transportation limitations. Collaboration between public transportation agencies, community organizations, and residents is key to developing effective and sustainable transportation strategies for food deserts.

Innovative Solutions for Improving Transportation in Food Deserts

Transportation barriers play a significant role in exacerbating food deserts, limiting individuals' access to healthy and affordable food options. Addressing these transportation challenges requires innovative solutions that can improve food access and promote equity. In this section, we will explore various strategies and interventions that have been implemented to enhance transportation in food desert areas.

Collaboration between Transportation and Food Systems

One approach to improving transportation in food deserts is to foster collaboration between transportation and food systems. By integrating these two sectors, it becomes possible to create innovative solutions that address the needs of both transportation and food access simultaneously.

For instance, public transportation systems can work together with local food retailers to establish dedicated bus routes that connect food deserts with grocery stores or farmers markets. These routes can be strategically planned, considering the location of food deserts and the availability of fresh and nutritious food sources. By coordinating schedules and routes, individuals living in food deserts can easily access grocery stores without relying on personal vehicles.

Another collaborative initiative is the establishment of mobile farmers markets or grocery stores. These vehicles bring fresh produce and other food items directly to underserved communities, eliminating the need for individuals to travel long distances to access healthy food options. Mobile markets can visit different neighborhoods on scheduled days, ensuring that residents have consistent access to a variety of nutritious foods.

Ridesharing and Carpooling Solutions

In areas where public transportation is limited, ridesharing and carpooling solutions can play a vital role in improving transportation options for individuals in food deserts. These innovative approaches leverage technology to connect drivers with passengers in need of transportation.

Ridesharing services, such as Uber or Lyft, can be utilized to provide individuals in food deserts with reliable transportation to grocery stores or supermarkets. By using smartphone applications, residents can request a ride and be connected with a driver who will take them to their desired destination. To address affordability concerns, subsidies or discounted fares can be provided for low-income individuals.

Carpooling initiatives also offer a viable transportation solution for communities affected by food deserts. By encouraging neighbors and community members to share rides to grocery stores, the cost and burden of transportation can be distributed among multiple individuals. Community organizations or local governments can establish carpooling programs, provide incentives, and facilitate connections between residents for effective implementation.

Bicycle and Pedestrian Infrastructure

Promoting active transportation options, such as walking and cycling, is another innovative solution for improving transportation in food deserts. Investing in bicycle and pedestrian infrastructure can create safe and accessible routes for individuals to reach grocery stores and farmers markets within their communities.

Building dedicated bike lanes, pedestrian-friendly sidewalks, and crosswalks can encourage residents to choose walking or cycling as their primary mode of transportation. These infrastructure improvements not only facilitate access to healthy food options but also promote physical activity, leading to improved health outcomes.

To further support active transportation, bike-sharing programs can be implemented in food desert areas. These programs provide affordable access to bicycles, allowing individuals to conveniently travel to grocery stores and other destinations. Partnerships with local businesses or non-profit organizations can offer reduced or subsidized bike-sharing memberships for low-income residents.

Online Ordering and Delivery Services

In the digital age, online ordering and delivery services have emerged as innovative solutions to overcome transportation barriers in food deserts. These services provide individuals with the convenience of ordering groceries or fresh produce online and having them delivered directly to their doorstep.

Online platforms or mobile applications can be developed specifically for food desert communities, featuring partnerships with local grocery stores or farmers markets. Residents can browse through a wide range of food items, select their desired products, and schedule a delivery that meets their needs. This approach eliminates the need for physical transportation to access healthy food options, ensuring convenience and promoting food security.

To address affordability concerns, subsidies or reduced delivery fees can be provided for individuals living in low-income areas. Additionally, community organizations or non-profit entities can collaborate with local food retailers to establish cooperative delivery programs, ensuring that residents have consistent access to affordable and nutritious food.

Conclusion

Transportation plays a crucial role in addressing food deserts and ensuring equitable access to healthy food options. In this section, we explored innovative solutions for improving transportation in food desert areas, including collaboration between transportation and food systems, ridesharing and carpooling solutions, bicycle and pedestrian infrastructure, and online ordering and delivery services. By implementing these strategies, communities can overcome transportation barriers and create a more inclusive food environment. However, it is important to note that these solutions should be tailored to the specific needs and contexts of each food desert, considering factors such as demographics, geography, and community preferences. Addressing transportation challenges in food deserts requires a comprehensive and multi-faceted approach that prioritizes equity, health, and sustainability.

Educational Attainment and Food Choices

Education and nutrition knowledge

Education plays a crucial role in shaping individuals' knowledge and understanding of proper nutrition. It provides the foundation for making informed choices about the food we consume and the impact it has on our health. In this section, we will explore the relationship between education and nutrition knowledge, highlighting the importance of education in promoting healthy food choices and addressing the challenges faced in food deserts.

The role of education in nutrition

Education is a key determinant of health outcomes, including nutrition. It equips individuals with the knowledge, skills, and resources necessary to make informed decisions about their dietary habits. A solid understanding of nutrition empowers individuals to choose healthier foods, avoid harmful dietary practices, and improve their overall well-being.

Formal education, such as school-based nutrition programs and educational curricula, provides a structured platform for imparting nutrition knowledge to children and adolescents. These programs can cover a wide range of topics, including the basics of nutrition, understanding food labels, meal planning, and the importance of balanced diets. By incorporating nutrition education into the curriculum, schools can promote healthy eating habits from an early age, setting the foundation for a lifetime of good nutrition.

In addition to formal education, informal sources of nutrition knowledge, such as media, community programs, and peer networks, also play a significant role. For example, television shows, websites, and social media platforms can disseminate information about healthy eating practices, recipes, and nutrition tips. Community programs and workshops can provide hands-on experiences and practical guidance on healthy cooking and eating habits. Peer networks and support groups can serve as important sources of information exchange and social support for individuals seeking to improve their nutrition.

Barriers to nutrition knowledge in food deserts

While education is an essential tool for promoting nutrition knowledge, individuals living in food deserts often face specific barriers that hinder their access to education and information about healthy eating. These barriers include:

- **Limited educational resources:** Schools and educational institutions in food deserts may lack adequate resources and funding to provide comprehensive nutrition education programs. This limitation can result in a lack of access to quality nutrition education for students in these areas.

- **Limited access to information:** Food deserts are often characterized by limited access to grocery stores and supermarkets, which also limits access to educational materials on nutrition. Without access to reliable sources of information, individuals may struggle to gain a deeper understanding of nutrition principles and healthy food choices.

- **Language and cultural barriers:** Some individuals living in food deserts may face language barriers, which can impede their understanding of nutrition education materials that are not provided in their native language. Cultural differences and traditional dietary practices can also impact the relevance and acceptance of nutrition knowledge in these communities.

- **Low health literacy:** Limited education and low health literacy levels among individuals in food deserts can present additional challenges. Poor health literacy hinders individuals' ability to understand and utilize health-related information effectively, including nutrition education materials.

Addressing the barriers to nutrition knowledge in food deserts requires a multi-faceted approach that takes into account the unique needs and challenges of these communities.

Innovations in nutrition education in food deserts

Efforts are underway to develop innovative approaches to nutrition education in food deserts. These initiatives aim to overcome the barriers mentioned earlier and provide accessible and culturally relevant nutrition education to individuals living in these areas. Here are a few examples of such innovations:

- **Mobile applications:** Mobile applications have gained popularity in recent years as a means of delivering nutrition education. These apps provide users with interactive tools, recipes, and informative content about healthy eating. They can be tailored to specific dietary needs, cultural preferences, and language requirements, making them a useful tool in addressing barriers such as limited access to educational resources and language/cultural differences.

- **Community-based nutrition programs:** Community-based nutrition programs leverage local resources and engage community members in promoting healthy eating habits. These programs can include cooking classes, workshops, and grocery store tours to increase nutrition knowledge and awareness. By involving residents in these programs, they can become active agents in spreading nutrition knowledge within their communities.

- **Peer education programs:** Peer education programs empower individuals with nutrition knowledge to serve as educators and advocates within their communities. Trained peer educators can deliver targeted nutrition education sessions, sharing information and practical tips with their peers about healthy eating habits and access to nutritious foods.

- **School-community partnerships:** Collaborations between schools and community organizations can enhance nutrition education efforts. By integrating community resources, such as local gardens or farmers markets, into the school curriculum, students can gain hands-on experience with nutritious food and learn about the importance of sustainable and locally sourced options.

These innovative approaches to nutrition education in food deserts aim to overcome the barriers posed by limited educational resources, lack of information access, language/cultural differences, and low health literacy levels. By implementing tailored and culturally appropriate strategies, individuals in food deserts can gain access to nutrition knowledge and improve their overall health and well-being.

Case study: The "Healthy Corner Store" program

One successful example of a nutrition education initiative in food deserts is the "Healthy Corner Store" program. This program aims to improve access to healthy food options and nutrition knowledge in underserved communities by working with small corner stores to increase the availability of fresh produce, whole grains, and low-fat dairy products.

In addition to improving the food options available, the program also provides nutrition education and training to store owners and staff. Store owners are educated on the benefits of stocking healthier foods, how to source and store fresh produce, and how to market these products effectively.

To enhance community engagement, the program also conducts nutrition workshops and cooking demonstrations in collaboration with local community organizations. These workshops provide residents with practical nutrition knowledge, meal planning tips, and cooking strategies using the healthier food options available in their local corner stores.

The "Healthy Corner Store" program is a holistic approach to addressing the lack of access to nutritious food and nutrition knowledge in food deserts. By working with the existing infrastructure of corner stores, this program creates sustainable solutions that address both the supply of healthy food options and the demand for nutrition education.

Conclusion

Education is a powerful tool in promoting nutrition knowledge and improving dietary habits. In food deserts, where access to healthy foods and educational resources is limited, targeted and innovative approaches are essential. By overcoming barriers such as limited resources, access to information, language/cultural differences, and low health literacy, individuals in food deserts can gain the necessary knowledge and skills to make informed choices about their nutrition.

Initiatives such as mobile applications, community-based programs, peer education, and school-community partnerships are paving the way for nutrition education in food deserts. These innovative approaches aim to bridge the gap in nutrition knowledge and empower communities to take control of their health and well-being.

In the next section, we will explore the impact of employment and food insecurity on nutrition in food deserts."

Impact of education on food preferences

Education plays a significant role in shaping an individual's food preferences. It provides knowledge and awareness about nutrition, which in turn influences the choices people make regarding the food they consume. In this section, we will explore how education impacts food preferences and how it can lead to healthier eating habits in individuals.

Education and nutrition knowledge

One of the main ways education influences food preferences is by imparting nutrition knowledge to individuals. Through educational programs, schools, and community initiatives, individuals gain a better understanding of the importance of a balanced diet and the role of different nutrients in promoting overall health and well-being. This knowledge equips individuals with the necessary information to make informed decisions about the foods they eat.

For example, educational initiatives can teach individuals about the nutritional value of fruits and vegetables, the benefits of whole grains, and the potential health risks associated with excessive intake of processed or sugary foods. Such knowledge can help individuals develop preferences for nutrient-dense foods and reduce their consumption of unhealthy options.

Impact of education on food preferences

Education has a direct impact on food preferences by shaping individuals' attitudes, beliefs, and values regarding food. When individuals are educated about the importance of a healthy diet, they are more likely to develop positive attitudes towards nutritious foods and prioritize them in their eating habits.

Studies have shown that individuals with higher levels of education tend to have a greater preference for healthier foods, such as fruits, vegetables, whole grains, and lean proteins. This can be attributed to their understanding of the nutritional benefits of these foods and their ability to make informed choices based on that knowledge.

Furthermore, education can influence individuals' taste preferences. As individuals learn about different flavor profiles, cooking techniques, and culinary traditions from various cultures, they become more open to trying new foods and expanding their palate. This exposure to diverse foods can lead to a broader range of food preferences and a greater willingness to experiment with healthier options.

Education and health literacy in food deserts

In the context of food deserts, where access to healthy foods is limited, education becomes even more crucial. It can serve as a tool to empower individuals living in food deserts to make healthier choices within the constraints of their environment.

Educational initiatives targeting food deserts can focus on providing information on alternative food sources, such as community gardens, farmers markets, or food cooperatives. By educating individuals about these options and their benefits, they can be encouraged to seek out and utilize these resources to access fresh, nutritious foods.

Furthermore, education can help individuals in food deserts develop skills in meal planning, food budgeting, and cooking with limited resources. These practical skills can enable them to make the most of the available food options and create healthier meals for themselves and their families.

Example: School-based nutrition education

A prime example of the impact of education on food preferences is school-based nutrition education programs. These programs aim to teach children about healthy eating habits and the importance of a balanced diet. By providing nutrition education at an early age, schools can help shape children's food preferences and establish a strong foundation for a lifetime of healthy eating.

School-based nutrition education can take various forms, such as interactive classroom sessions, cooking demonstrations, and involvement in school gardens. By engaging children in hands-on activities, they learn about different food groups, the benefits of making healthy choices, and how to prepare nutritious meals.

Research has shown that school-based nutrition education programs can have a positive impact on children's food preferences. Children who participate in these programs are more likely to consume fruits and vegetables, choose whole grains over refined grains, and opt for healthier snacks. This demonstrates the power of education in influencing food preferences and promoting healthier eating habits from a young age.

Conclusion

In conclusion, education plays a crucial role in shaping individuals' food preferences. By providing nutrition knowledge, it empowers individuals to make informed choices about the foods they consume. Education also influences attitudes, beliefs, and taste preferences related to food, leading to a greater preference for healthier options. In the context of food deserts, education becomes a vital tool for promoting health literacy and empowering individuals to navigate their food environment effectively. Through school-based nutrition education programs and other initiatives, education can have a significant positive impact on individuals' food preferences and contribute to overall improvements in nutrition and health.

Education and health literacy in food deserts

Food deserts not only restrict access to nutritious food, but they also present challenges in terms of education and health literacy. In this section, we will explore the impact of education on food choices, the role of education in improving health literacy, and the challenges faced by individuals living in food deserts in acquiring this knowledge.

Education and nutrition knowledge

Education plays a crucial role in shaping individuals' understanding of nutrition and food choices. Those with higher levels of education generally have better knowledge about healthy diets and are more likely to make informed food choices. However, in food deserts, educational attainment is often lower compared to other areas, creating a knowledge gap that perpetuates poor eating habits.

Limited access to quality education can hinder individuals' ability to understand the importance of a healthy diet and make informed food choices. Schools in food desert areas may lack the resources to provide comprehensive nutrition education, leading to a lack of awareness about the importance of healthy food. As a result, individuals may rely on cheap, processed, and unhealthy foods available in their neighborhoods.

Impact of education on food preferences

Research has shown that education has a significant impact on individuals' food preferences. Education equips individuals with knowledge about the nutritional value of various foods, the impact of diet on health, and the importance of consuming a balanced diet. This knowledge can influence food preferences and lead to the adoption of healthier eating habits.

Individuals with higher levels of education are more likely to have access to a wide range of information sources, such as scientific research, nutrition education programs, and cooking classes. This exposure allows them to develop a deeper understanding of the benefits of consuming fresh fruits and vegetables, whole grains, and lean proteins. As a result, they are more likely to incorporate these foods into their diets.

Conversely, individuals with limited education may lack the necessary knowledge to make healthy food choices. They may not be aware of the negative health consequences associated with consuming processed and fast foods regularly. Additionally, they may face financial constraints that limit their access to nutritious foods, further exacerbating the problem.

Education and health literacy in food deserts

Health literacy refers to an individual's ability to access, understand, and apply health-related information and services to make informed decisions. In food deserts, limited access to quality education can negatively impact health literacy levels, making it difficult for individuals to navigate health information and make informed decisions about their dietary choices.

Living in a food desert can restrict individuals' exposure to health information and resources. Limited access to supermarkets and grocery stores means that individuals may not have access to nutrition labels, dietary guidelines, or educational materials that can help them make healthier choices. They may also lack the knowledge to interpret and apply the information they do have access to, further limiting their ability to improve their health.

Moreover, individuals living in food deserts may face additional barriers to acquiring health literacy, such as language barriers, low literacy rates, and limited digital literacy. These barriers can make it challenging to access and understand health resources, exacerbating the negative impact of food deserts on health outcomes.

Addressing the issue of health literacy in food deserts requires a multi-faceted approach. Providing comprehensive nutrition education in schools, community centers, and healthcare facilities can equip individuals with the knowledge and skills needed to make healthier food choices. Additionally, programs that promote digital and media literacy can empower individuals to access and critically evaluate health information from various sources.

Example: Nutrition education initiatives in food deserts

To illustrate the importance of education and health literacy in food deserts, let's consider an example of a successful nutrition education initiative.

The "Healthy Food, Healthy Lives" program was implemented in a food desert community with limited access to fresh and nutritious foods. The program aimed to educate residents about the benefits of a healthy diet and provide practical skills to make healthier food choices.

The initiative involved partnering with local schools to incorporate nutrition education into the curriculum. Students received lessons on various topics, such as understanding food labels, identifying healthy food options, and preparing simple and nutritious meals. The program also organized cooking workshops and grocery store tours to enhance practical skills and expose students to healthier food options.

In addition to school-based initiatives, community workshops were organized to extend nutrition education to adults. These workshops covered a range of topics, including meal planning, budgeting for healthy food, and strategies for overcoming barriers to healthy eating. The program also collaborated with local healthcare providers to offer free nutrition counseling services to community members.

Evaluation of the program showed significant improvements in nutrition knowledge, dietary habits, and health outcomes among participants. Participants reported increased confidence in making healthier food choices and demonstrated improved dietary diversity. The initiative's success can be attributed to its comprehensive approach, combining education, practical skills development, and community engagement.

Caveats and challenges

While education and health literacy are crucial in addressing the impact of food deserts, there are several challenges that need to be considered:

- Limited resources: Schools and community organizations in food deserts may have limited resources to provide comprehensive nutrition education. Funding constraints and lack of trained educators can hinder the implementation of effective programs.

- Cultural factors: Education and health promotion efforts need to consider cultural differences and tailor interventions accordingly. Cultural beliefs and practices related to food can influence dietary choices, and educational programs should be culturally sensitive and inclusive.

- Limited access to information: Even with proper education, individuals in food deserts may still face challenges in accessing accurate and reliable health information. Addressing the digital divide and ensuring the availability of health resources in various formats is essential.

Overcoming these challenges requires collaborative efforts between educators, healthcare providers, community organizations, and policymakers. By addressing the limitations and investing in education and health literacy initiatives, we can empower individuals living in food deserts to make healthier choices and improve their overall well-being.

Summary

In this section, we explored the impact of education and health literacy in food deserts. We discussed how limited access to quality education can contribute to poor nutrition knowledge and unhealthy food preferences. We highlighted the role of education in improving health literacy and the challenges faced by individuals in acquiring this knowledge in food deserts.

Additionally, we provided an example of a successful nutrition education initiative implemented in a food desert community. We emphasized the importance of comprehensive approaches that combine education, practical skills development, and community engagement to drive positive changes in dietary habits and health outcomes.

However, we acknowledged the caveats and challenges that exist in addressing education and health literacy in food deserts, such as limited resources, cultural factors, and access to information. These challenges need to be considered and addressed through collaborative efforts to ensure equitable access to education and improve health outcomes in food deserts.

Employment and Food Insecurity

Employment Opportunities in Food Deserts

The lack of employment opportunities in food deserts exacerbates the challenges faced by individuals living in these communities. Limited job prospects contribute to low income levels and high rates of poverty, which further restrict access to healthy and affordable food options. In this section, we will explore the various socioeconomic factors that contribute to the dearth of employment opportunities in food deserts and discuss potential solutions to address this issue.

Poverty and Unemployment Rates

In food deserts, poverty rates tend to be higher than the national average. This lack of economic resources hinders individuals' ability to afford nutritious food and perpetuates a cycle of food insecurity. Furthermore, high levels of poverty are closely linked to high unemployment rates.

Example: In the urban food desert of East Harlem in New York City, the poverty rate is approximately 30

Limited Job Market

One of the key contributors to the limited employment opportunities in food deserts is the absence of a diverse and robust job market. Factors such as lack of local businesses, inadequate transportation infrastructure, and the concentration of low-income residents in these areas contribute to the scarcity of jobs.

Example: In rural food deserts, the sparse population and geographic isolation make it difficult for businesses to thrive. As a result, job opportunities are limited, and residents often have to travel long distances to access employment.

Low-skilled and Low-wage Jobs

In many food deserts, the available employment opportunities are often low-skilled and low-wage jobs. This can be attributed to a combination of factors, including the lack of educational resources, limited job training programs, and the absence of industries that offer higher-paying positions.

Example: In some urban food deserts, the most common jobs available are in the service industry, such as fast-food restaurants and convenience stores. These jobs typically offer low wages and limited opportunities for career advancement.

Solutions and Interventions

Addressing the lack of employment opportunities in food deserts requires a comprehensive approach that takes into account the unique challenges faced by these communities. Some potential solutions and interventions are:

1. **Job Creation Programs:** Government-funded programs can be implemented to create job opportunities in food deserts. These programs could involve infrastructure projects, green initiatives, or the establishment of cooperatives and social enterprises.

2. **Entrepreneurship Support:** Providing support and resources for individuals interested in starting their own businesses in food deserts can help stimulate the local economy and create job opportunities. This could include access to loans, business training programs, and mentorship.

3. **Workforce Development Initiatives:** Investing in workforce development programs that target specific skills needed in the local job market can help residents gain the necessary qualifications for employment. These programs could offer vocational training, job placement assistance, and apprenticeship opportunities.

4. **Public-Private Partnerships:** Collaboration between the government, private sector, and community organizations can help attract businesses to food deserts and create sustainable job opportunities. Incentives such as tax breaks, grants, and support for local entrepreneurs can be provided to encourage investment in these communities.

Addressing Systemic Barriers

It is important to recognize that addressing the lack of employment opportunities in food deserts requires a multi-dimensional approach that not only focuses on creating job opportunities but also tackles systemic barriers that contribute to economic inequality. These systemic barriers include discriminatory hiring practices, unequal access to quality education, and limited resources for skill development.

Example: Implementing policies that promote equal opportunity employment, improve access to education and vocational training, and provide support for underrepresented individuals can help break down systemic barriers and create a more inclusive job market in food deserts.

Building Sustainable Local Economies

Creating sustainable local economies in food deserts is crucial for long-term economic growth and job creation. This can be achieved through strategies such as:

1. **Supporting Local Businesses:** Investing in local businesses, particularly those that provide healthy food options, can help stimulate economic growth in food deserts. This can be done through financial support, technical assistance, and marketing initiatives.

2. **Promoting Community Ownership:** Encouraging community ownership of businesses through cooperative models or community development corporations can help ensure that economic benefits stay within the local community, creating a more resilient and sustainable economy.

3. **Fostering Entrepreneurship:** Providing resources and support for aspiring entrepreneurs in food deserts can help them start and grow their businesses. This includes access to capital, mentorship programs, and business incubators.

Conclusion

The lack of employment opportunities in food deserts contributes to the cycle of poverty and limited access to healthy food. Addressing this issue requires a multi-faceted approach that includes job creation programs, entrepreneurship support, workforce development initiatives, and the dismantling of systemic barriers. By building sustainable local economies and promoting inclusive employment practices, we can help break the cycle of food insecurity and create healthier and thriving communities.

Income Instability and Food Insecurity

Income instability and food insecurity are closely intertwined issues that significantly contribute to the existence and persistence of food deserts. In this section, we will explore the relationship between income instability, food insecurity, and their impact on access to healthy food options in food deserts. We will also discuss the consequences of inadequate income and food access on individuals and communities, as well as explore potential solutions to address these challenges.

Understanding Income Instability

Income instability refers to the irregularity or unpredictability of income, which can be attributed to various factors such as fluctuations in employment, changes in work hours, or economic downturns. Individuals and families experiencing income instability often face difficulties in managing their financial resources, leading to challenges in meeting basic needs, including accessing affordable and nutritious food.

One major consequence of income instability is the inability to consistently afford an adequate amount of food, which is known as food insecurity. A person or household is considered food insecure when they have limited or uncertain access to sufficient, safe, and nutritious food to meet their dietary needs and preferences for an active and healthy life.

The Link between Income Instability and Food Insecurity

Income instability and food insecurity are interconnected, exacerbating each other's effects. When individuals experience income instability, it becomes challenging to plan and budget for daily expenses, including food. Fluctuating incomes can make it difficult to consistently afford healthy food options, forcing individuals to rely on cheaper, unhealthy alternatives. This leads to compromised nutrition and negative health outcomes, including an increased risk of diet-related diseases like obesity, diabetes, and heart disease.

Moreover, the uncertainty associated with income instability can create anxiety and stress, further impacting individuals' mental well-being. Mental health issues can affect their ability to make informed decisions regarding food choices, leading to a higher likelihood of opting for cheaper, processed, and unhealthy food options.

Implications of Income Instability and Food Insecurity in Food Deserts

In food desert communities, income instability and food insecurity pose even greater challenges. Limited access to affordable and nutritious food options already characterizes food deserts, and income instability exacerbates this problem. Low-income individuals living in food deserts are more likely to experience fluctuations in income due to precarious employment opportunities, such as part-time or seasonal work. This income volatility makes it even more challenging for them to consistently afford healthy food choices.

Food insecurity resulting from income instability not only affects individuals' nutritional well-being but also has broader implications for community health. Inadequate nutrition can undermine overall health, leading to higher healthcare costs, decreased productivity, and diminished quality of life. Moreover, food insecurity can perpetuate cycles of poverty, as individuals and families struggling with inadequate access to food may find it difficult to improve their economic circumstances.

Addressing Income Instability and Food Insecurity

Addressing income instability and food insecurity requires a multi-faceted approach that combines economic, social, and policy interventions. Here are some potential strategies to mitigate these issues:

- **Livelihood Support Programs:** Providing stable employment opportunities, skills training, and income support programs can help reduce income instability among vulnerable populations.

- **Minimum Wage Policies:** Implementing fair minimum wage policies can ensure a more stable income for low-wage workers, reducing income volatility and enhancing their ability to afford nutritious food.

- **Social Safety Nets:** Establishing and strengthening social safety net programs, such as unemployment benefits, food assistance programs, and cash transfer schemes, can help buffer the impact of income shocks and ensure access to adequate food during periods of instability.

- **Education and Financial Literacy:** Promoting financial literacy programs can empower individuals to better manage their income and allocate resources towards nutritional priorities, even during periods of income instability.

- **Community Initiatives:** Encouraging community-based solutions, such as food cooperatives, community gardens, and food sharing networks, can enhance food security by increasing access to affordable, nutritious food within food desert neighborhoods.

By addressing income instability and food insecurity together, policymakers, community leaders, and individuals can work towards sustainable solutions that improve access to healthy food options, promote social justice, and foster healthier communities.

Summary

In this section, we explored the relationship between income instability and food insecurity in the context of food deserts. Income instability can significantly impact individuals' ability to afford healthy food options, leading to food insecurity. This issue is particularly prevalent in food desert communities, where access to affordable and nutritious food is already limited. We discussed the implications of income instability and food insecurity on individuals' health and well-being, highlighting the need for comprehensive strategies to address these challenges. By implementing measures such as livelihood support programs, minimum wage policies, social safety nets, education, and community initiatives, we can begin to mitigate income instability and food insecurity in food deserts, fostering more equitable access to healthy food and promoting overall community well-being.

Government Assistance Programs and Food Access

Government assistance programs play a crucial role in addressing food access issues in food deserts. These programs aim to provide support and resources to individuals and families who struggle to obtain nutritious food. In this section, we will explore the various government assistance programs and initiatives that have been implemented to improve food access in food deserts.

Supplemental Nutrition Assistance Program (SNAP)

The Supplemental Nutrition Assistance Program (SNAP) is one of the most significant government assistance programs in the United States. Formerly known as food stamps, SNAP provides eligible low-income individuals and families with electronic benefit transfer cards that can be used to purchase food items from authorized retailers.

SNAP benefits are determined based on household size, income, and expenses. Participants can use their SNAP benefits to buy a wide range of food items, including fruits, vegetables, meat, dairy products, grains, and non-alcoholic beverages. However, certain items like tobacco, alcohol, and hot prepared foods are not eligible for purchase with SNAP benefits.

The impact of SNAP on food access in food deserts has been significant. Studies have shown that SNAP participation is associated with increased consumption of fruits and vegetables among low-income individuals. Additionally, SNAP benefits have been found to reduce the prevalence of food insecurity and improve dietary quality among participants.

WIC Program

The Special Supplemental Nutrition Program for Women, Infants, and Children (WIC) is another important government assistance program that focuses on improving the nutritional status of pregnant, postpartum, and breastfeeding women, as well as infants and children up to age five. WIC provides eligible participants with vouchers that can be used to purchase specific nutritious food items, including fruits, vegetables, whole grains, dairy products, and infant formula.

In addition to providing nutritious food, the WIC program also offers nutrition education, counseling, and support to participants. This comprehensive approach aims to promote healthy eating behaviors and improve long-term health outcomes.

The WIC program has been successful in increasing the consumption of essential nutrients among women and children from low-income households. Studies have shown that WIC participants have higher intakes of key nutrients, such as iron, calcium, and vitamin C, compared to non-participants.

School Meal Programs

School meal programs, including the National School Lunch Program (NSLP) and the School Breakfast Program (SBP), are crucial in ensuring that children from low-income families have access to nutritious meals during the school day.

The NSLP provides free or reduced-price lunches to eligible students, while the SBP ensures that children have access to a healthy breakfast before school. These programs not only help alleviate immediate hunger but also contribute to better overall nutrition and academic performance.

To further support food access in food deserts, some schools have implemented innovative initiatives such as the Community Eligibility Provision (CEP). The CEP allows schools in low-income areas to offer free meals to all students, regardless of income, eliminating barriers to access and ensuring that no child goes hungry.

Senior Nutrition Programs

Senior nutrition programs aim to address the specific nutritional needs of older adults, many of whom live in food deserts and face challenges in accessing nutritious food. The Older Americans Act Nutrition Program, for example, provides congregate and home-delivered meals to older adults, ensuring that they receive adequate nutrition.

In addition to meal provision, senior nutrition programs often offer nutrition education, health screenings, and socialization opportunities for seniors. These programs play a crucial role in improving the health and well-being of older adults in food deserts.

Addressing Challenges and Improving Effectiveness

While government assistance programs have made significant strides in improving food access in food deserts, several challenges persist. Limited program funding, administrative barriers, and stigma associated with receiving assistance can hinder participation and effectiveness.

To address these challenges, ongoing efforts are being made to streamline program enrollment processes, increase program outreach and education, and reduce stigma. Additionally, advocacy and policy changes are necessary to ensure that government assistance programs have adequate funding to meet the needs of individuals and families in food deserts.

Community partnerships and collaborations also play a vital role in improving the effectiveness of government assistance programs. By working together with community organizations, nonprofit agencies, and local businesses, government programs can leverage additional resources and reach a broader audience.

Moreover, continuous evaluation and monitoring of program outcomes are crucial in identifying areas for improvement and ensuring that resources are allocated effectively. By collecting data on food access, nutritional outcomes, and participant satisfaction, policymakers can make informed decisions and implement evidence-based strategies.

Overall, government assistance programs are indispensable in addressing food access issues in food deserts. By providing resources, education, and support, these programs strive to empower individuals and communities to make healthier food choices and improve their overall well-being. However, ongoing efforts are needed to overcome challenges and ensure equitable access to nutritious food for all.

Race and Ethnicity in Food Deserts

Racial Disparities in Food Access

Racial disparities in food access refer to the unequal distribution of healthy and affordable food based on racial or ethnic backgrounds. These disparities are rooted in historical and socio-cultural factors, as well as systemic inequalities. This section explores the various dimensions of racial disparities in food access, their causes, and potential strategies to address them.

Historical and Socio-Cultural Factors

The historical context plays a significant role in understanding racial disparities in food access. Historical events such as segregation, redlining, and discriminatory urban planning have resulted in the concentration of racial minority populations in low-income neighborhoods with limited access to fresh and nutritious food. These neighborhoods, often referred to as food deserts, lack grocery stores and farmers markets, and instead are inundated with fast food restaurants and convenience stores that offer predominantly unhealthy food options.

Socio-cultural factors also contribute to racial disparities in food access. Cultural food preferences, traditions, and dietary practices can influence the availability and affordability of certain types of food in specific communities. Discrimination and prejudice in the food industry can further exacerbate these disparities, making it harder for racial minorities to access quality food options.

Structural Inequalities

Structural inequalities, such as income disparities, lack of economic opportunities, and limited access to transportation, significantly contribute to racial disparities in food access. Many racial minority communities face higher levels of poverty and unemployment, making it difficult to afford nutritious food. The lack of well-paying jobs and economic opportunities result in limited resources for food purchases, leaving individuals and families with no choice but to rely on cheaper, processed foods that are often high in added sugars, unhealthy fats, and sodium.

Additionally, racial disparities in transportation access compound the problem. Many low-income neighborhoods, predominantly inhabited by racial minorities, lack reliable and affordable transportation options. This limits their ability to travel to areas with better food retail options, leaving them dependent on what is available within their immediate vicinity.

Environmental Racism

Environmental racism, the disproportionate burden of environmental hazards on racial minority communities, also contributes to racial disparities in food access. Food deserts are often located in areas with higher levels of environmental pollution and limited green spaces. These neighborhoods may have contaminated soil, making it difficult to establish community gardens or urban farms. As a result, the availability of fresh, locally-grown produce is limited in these areas, forcing residents to rely on processed and unhealthy food options.

Addressing Racial Inequalities in Food Deserts

Addressing racial disparities in food access requires a comprehensive and multi-pronged approach. Here are some strategies and interventions that have shown promise:

1. Promoting Equitable Food Retail: Encouraging the establishment of grocery stores, farmers markets, and community gardens in food deserts helps increase access to fresh and healthy food. Incentives, subsidies, and zoning changes can attract food retailers to underserved neighborhoods.
2. Transportation Solutions: Improving transportation infrastructure, expanding public transit options, and providing discounted or free transportation services specifically for accessing food retail can address transportation barriers in food deserts, particularly in racially marginalized areas.
3. Community Empowerment: Engaging and empowering local communities through education and capacity-building initiatives can help them advocate for their own food security. Supporting community-led initiatives, such as community gardens and urban farming programs, fosters self-reliance and promotes sustainable food access.
4. Policy and Legislation: Implementing policies and legislation that address systemic issues contributing to racial disparities in food access is crucial. This includes promoting equitable land-use policies, increasing funding for nutrition assistance programs, and addressing discriminatory practices in the food industry.
5. Education and Health Promotion: Investing in nutrition education programs, cooking classes, and health promotion campaigns tailored to racial minority communities can enhance their knowledge and skills related to healthy

food choices. Empowering individuals with the information they need to make informed decisions fosters long-term behavior change.

6. Collaboration and Partnerships: Collaboration between government agencies, non-profit organizations, community groups, and businesses is essential to address racial disparities in food access holistically. Building strategic partnerships can leverage resources and expertise to develop comprehensive interventions and ensure their sustainability.

Example: The Healthy Food Financing Initiative

An example of a policy initiative aimed at tackling racial disparities in food access is the Healthy Food Financing Initiative (HFFI). The HFFI, launched by the U.S. Department of Agriculture, seeks to improve access to healthy food in underserved communities, including food deserts with a high proportion of racial minorities.

The HFFI provides financial support and tax incentives for businesses and organizations to establish grocery stores and other fresh food retail outlets in areas with limited access to healthy food options. By incentivizing food retailers to invest in underserved communities, the initiative creates opportunities for racial minorities to access quality food closer to their homes.

The HFFI also emphasizes community engagement and partnership by requiring funded projects to include community input in their planning and design phases. This approach ensures that interventions are tailored to address the specific needs of racial minority communities and encourages community ownership and empowerment.

Conclusion

Racial disparities in food access are deeply interconnected with historical, structural, and socio-cultural factors. Addressing these disparities requires a comprehensive approach that tackles systemic inequalities, promotes community-driven solutions, and advocates for policy changes. By implementing strategies aimed at improving food access, reducing environmental racism, and empowering racial minority communities, we can work towards a more equitable and just food system for all.

Historical and Socio-Cultural Factors

Historical and socio-cultural factors play a significant role in understanding the origins and perpetuation of food deserts. These factors shape the social and economic landscape, which ultimately affects the availability and accessibility of healthy food options in certain communities. By examining historical and socio-cultural factors, we can gain insight into the root causes of food deserts and develop effective strategies to address them.

Historical Context

To understand the historical factors contributing to food deserts, we must examine the broader context in which they emerged. One important historical factor is the phenomenon of urbanization. During the industrial revolution, there was a mass migration of people from rural areas to urban centers in search of better job opportunities. This rapid urbanization led to the growth of densely populated cities, where access to fresh and nutritious food became a challenge.

Another historical factor is racial segregation and discriminatory policies. In the United States, for example, the legacy of racial segregation and discriminatory practices such as redlining has had a profound impact on the spatial distribution of food resources. African American and minority communities, historically marginalized and economically disadvantaged by unfair policies, have been disproportionately affected by the lack of access to healthy food options.

Socio-Cultural Factors

In addition to historical factors, socio-cultural factors play a crucial role in shaping food deserts. Socio-cultural norms, beliefs, and practices influence food preferences, shopping habits, and dietary choices in a community. These factors can contribute to the limited availability of healthy food options and the prevalence of fast food or convenience stores in food deserts.

Cultural preferences and dietary traditions can influence the types of foods available in a particular area. In some communities, cultural norms may prioritize traditional foods that are not readily available in mainstream supermarkets, leading to limited access to culturally appropriate, healthy food options.

Furthermore, socio-economic inequalities, including income disparities, affect the ability of individuals and families to afford nutritious foods. Low-income communities often face financial constraints that make it difficult to purchase fresh produce or healthier food options, leading to a reliance on inexpensive, processed foods. This financial barrier perpetuates the cycle of limited access to healthy foods in food desert communities.

Examples and Case Studies

To illustrate the influence of historical and socio-cultural factors on food deserts, let's examine a few examples. In the United States, neighborhoods like the South Bronx in New York City and West Oakland in California have a long history of economic inequality, racial segregation, and limited access to fresh food. These communities have been negatively impacted by discriminatory housing practices, lack of investment, and a scarcity of supermarkets.

Internationally, the case of Glasgow, Scotland provides an insightful example. The city experienced deindustrialization in the 20th century, leading to high unemployment rates and poverty in certain areas. These deprived neighborhoods, often marked by a lack of grocery stores, have limited access to fresh and affordable food options.

These examples demonstrate that historical and socio-cultural factors are crucial in understanding the complex dynamics of food deserts. By acknowledging these factors and their impact, we can develop targeted interventions and policies to address the underlying causes of food deserts.

Addressing Historical and Socio-Cultural Factors

Addressing the historical and socio-cultural factors contributing to food deserts requires a multi-faceted approach. It involves recognizing the historical injustices and structural inequalities that have shaped these communities and developing strategies to address them. Here are some key steps:

1. Policy Changes: Implementing policies that promote equitable access to healthy food options is crucial. This includes initiatives such as zoning regulations to encourage the establishment of grocery stores in underserved areas, financial incentives for supermarkets to locate in food deserts, and expansion of public transportation networks to improve access to food retailers.

2. Community Engagement: Empowering local communities through participatory approaches is essential. Engaging community members in decision-making processes, such as the establishment of community gardens or farmers markets, can help ensure that interventions are culturally appropriate and meet the needs of the residents.

3. Education and Awareness: Promoting nutrition education and raising awareness about healthy food choices are vital components of addressing socio-cultural factors. By providing individuals with the knowledge and skills to make informed decisions about their food choices, we can empower them to overcome cultural barriers and adopt healthier lifestyles.

4. Addressing Inequalities: Tackling the root causes of food deserts requires addressing broader social and economic inequalities. This involves advocating for affordable housing, job opportunities, and income equality, as well as dismantling systemic racism and discrimination.

By considering historical and socio-cultural factors in tandem with other economic and geographical factors, we can gain a more comprehensive understanding of food deserts and develop effective interventions to eliminate them.

Key Takeaways

- Historical factors such as urbanization and racial segregation have contributed to the emergence of food deserts. - Socio-cultural factors, including cultural preferences and socio-economic inequalities, shape the availability and accessibility of healthy food in certain communities. - Examples of historically and socio-culturally influenced food deserts include neighborhoods in the United States like the South Bronx and West Oakland, as well as deprived areas in Glasgow, Scotland. - Addressing historical and socio-cultural factors requires policy changes, community engagement, education and awareness, and a focus on addressing broader social and economic inequalities. - Developing interventions that acknowledge historical and socio-cultural factors is essential for creating sustainable solutions to eliminate food deserts.

Addressing racial inequalities in food deserts

Addressing racial inequalities in food deserts is of utmost importance in achieving food justice and ensuring equitable access to healthy food for all communities. Racial disparities in food access have deep historical roots and are intertwined with broader social and economic inequalities. In this section, we will explore various strategies and interventions that can help address these racial inequalities and promote food equity in food desert neighborhoods.

Community engagement and empowerment

One of the key approaches to addressing racial inequalities in food deserts is through community engagement and empowerment. It is essential to involve the residents of these communities in decision-making processes and in shaping the solutions that can work best for them. By actively involving community members, their voices can be heard, and their unique needs and perspectives can be taken into account.

Community-led initiatives such as community gardens, urban farming, and farmers markets can play a vital role in addressing racial inequalities. These initiatives provide opportunities for residents, especially those from marginalized racial and ethnic groups, to grow their own food, have a direct market for fresh produce, and build sustainable local food systems. They not only increase food access but also create economic opportunities and empower individuals and communities.

Policy advocacy and legislation

Another critical aspect of addressing racial inequalities in food deserts is through policy advocacy and legislation. Advocacy groups, nonprofits, and community organizations can work together to push for policies that address the root causes of food deserts, including racial disparities in access to healthy food.

Policy changes can involve measures such as incentivizing grocery stores and supermarkets to open in underserved communities, implementing zoning regulations that support the establishment of food retail businesses, and providing financial assistance to small businesses and entrepreneurs from marginalized communities to start food retail ventures.

Additionally, legislation can focus on ensuring that healthy food options are available in schools and other public institutions in food desert neighborhoods, as well as improving the quality and affordability of meals provided through government assistance programs like school lunch programs and SNAP (Supplemental Nutrition Assistance Program).

Equitable food financing

Access to capital and financial resources is often a significant barrier for individuals and businesses in marginalized communities, particularly those owned by racial and ethnic minorities. Therefore, promoting equitable food financing is essential to address racial inequalities in food deserts.

Initiatives such as community development financial institutions (CDFIs) and microfinance programs can provide loans, grants, and technical assistance to aspiring entrepreneurs from disadvantaged backgrounds. By providing financial support and mentorship, these programs can help overcome the financial barriers faced by individuals and businesses in marginalized communities, allowing them to establish and maintain grocery stores, farmers markets, and other food retail enterprises.

Cultural relevance and education

Addressing racial inequalities in food deserts requires recognizing and respecting the cultural diversity of the communities affected. Food interventions should be culturally relevant, taking into account the unique food preferences, culinary traditions, and dietary practices of different racial and ethnic groups.

Efforts should be made to educate community members about nutrition and healthy eating practices, while also honoring and valuing their cultural food traditions. This can involve promoting culturally appropriate nutrition education programs, incorporating traditional foods into public school meals, and supporting local farmers who grow culturally significant crops.

Partnerships and collaborations

Collaborative efforts between various stakeholders, including government agencies, nonprofit organizations, community leaders, and businesses, are crucial in addressing racial inequalities in food deserts. Partnerships can pool resources, expertise, and knowledge to develop comprehensive and sustainable solutions.

These collaborations can involve establishing food policy councils or task forces that bring together representatives from diverse backgrounds to develop and implement strategies to address food inequities. It can also include forming alliances with healthcare providers, educational institutions, and local grassroots organizations to coordinate efforts and share resources.

Data collection and research

To effectively address racial inequalities in food deserts, it is essential to collect and analyze data on food access, health outcomes, and socioeconomic indicators within different racial and ethnic communities. This data can help identify the specific needs and challenges faced by different groups, inform targeted interventions, and measure the impact of various programs and policies.

Research should also focus on the intersectionality of race with other factors such as gender, socioeconomic status, and geographic location, to better understand the complexities of food deserts and develop tailored interventions.

Case study: The Healthy Food Financing Initiative

The Healthy Food Financing Initiative (HFFI) is an example of a national policy aimed at addressing racial inequalities in food deserts. This initiative, launched in

2010, provides financial support and technical assistance to grocery stores, farmers markets, and other food retail businesses in underserved communities.

Through grants and low-interest loans, the HFFI has helped fund the development and expansion of grocery stores in areas with limited access to healthy food, including many predominantly Black and Latino neighborhoods. The initiative has not only improved food access but also created employment opportunities within these communities.

The success of the HFFI highlights the importance of targeted policy interventions that address racial disparities in food access and promote economic development in marginalized communities.

Conclusion

Addressing racial inequalities in food deserts is a multifaceted challenge that requires comprehensive strategies and interventions. By actively involving communities, advocating for policy changes, promoting equitable food financing, recognizing cultural diversity, fostering partnerships, and conducting research, we can work towards achieving food justice and ensuring that all individuals, regardless of race or ethnicity, have access to fresh, healthy, and affordable food.

In the next section, we will delve into the health impacts of food deserts and explore how inadequate access to healthy food can adversely affect individuals and communities.

Health Impacts of Food Deserts

Nutritional Deficiencies and Health Risks

Lack of fresh produce and vitamins

Access to fresh produce and vitamins is a crucial aspect of a healthy diet. Unfortunately, food deserts often lack grocery stores or supermarkets that offer a wide variety of fresh fruits, vegetables, and other nutritious foods. As a result, individuals living in food deserts may experience a lack of fresh produce and vitamins in their diets, which can have significant health implications.

Fresh produce is an important source of essential vitamins, minerals, and fiber. Fruits and vegetables are rich in vitamins A, C, and E, as well as minerals like potassium, magnesium, and folate. These nutrients are vital for maintaining good health and preventing chronic diseases. For example, vitamin C supports a strong immune system and aids in wound healing, while vitamin A is crucial for maintaining healthy skin, vision, and immune function.

In a food desert, the absence of grocery stores with fresh produce options limits the availability of these important nutrients. This can lead to deficiencies in key vitamins and minerals, which can have a range of health consequences. For instance, inadequate intake of vitamin C can weaken the immune system, making individuals more susceptible to infections. Insufficient vitamin A intake can lead to vision problems and impaired immune function. Iron deficiency, commonly found in individuals with limited access to fresh produce, can result in anemia and fatigue.

Moreover, the lack of fresh produce can contribute to a higher intake of processed and unhealthy foods in food deserts. These foods are often high in calories, unhealthy fats, sodium, and added sugars but low in essential nutrients. Over time, a diet lacking in fresh produce and vitamins can increase the risk of various chronic diseases, including heart disease, obesity, and type 2 diabetes.

Addressing the lack of fresh produce and vitamins in food deserts requires a multifaceted approach. Here are some potential solutions:

1. Improve transportation options: Enhancing the availability and affordability of transportation can help individuals living in food deserts access grocery stores or farmers markets outside their immediate neighborhoods. This would increase their access to fresh produce.

2. Increase the number of farmer's markets: Farmer's markets offer a direct link between local farmers and consumers, providing an opportunity for individuals to access fresh, locally sourced produce. Supporting and expanding the number of farmer's markets in food deserts can help improve access to fresh fruits and vegetables.

3. Promote urban farming and community gardens: Creating spaces for urban farming and community gardens within food deserts can empower communities to grow their own fresh produce. This not only increases access but also promotes community engagement and education about healthy eating.

4. Provide financial incentives: Offering financial incentives, such as subsidies or tax breaks, to grocery stores and supermarkets that open in food deserts can encourage their establishment. This can improve the availability of fresh produce and increase competition, resulting in more affordable options for residents.

5. Educate and promote nutrition awareness: Implementing nutrition education programs targeted at food desert communities can empower individuals to make healthier food choices even with limited resources. This includes raising awareness about the importance of fresh produce and vitamins in a balanced diet.

By addressing the lack of fresh produce and vitamins in food deserts, we can improve the overall nutrition and health outcomes of individuals living in these areas. It is imperative to take a comprehensive approach that involves collaboration between government, community organizations, and individuals to create sustainable solutions for a healthier future.

Examples

Let's consider an example to illustrate the impact of the lack of fresh produce and vitamins on health.

Imagine a neighborhood that is classified as a food desert, with no accessible grocery stores offering fresh produce within a reasonable distance. The residents heavily rely on convenience stores and fast-food establishments, which typically have limited fresh produce options. As a result, their diets consist primarily of processed foods high in calories, unhealthy fats, and added sugars.

Over time, the lack of fresh produce and vitamins in their diets takes a toll on their health. Many individuals in the community develop obesity, type 2 diabetes, and heart disease due to poor dietary choices. The absence of essential vitamins and minerals further exacerbates these health conditions, making them more susceptible to infections and slower wound healing.

To address this issue, a grassroots organization in the neighborhood establishes a community garden. Residents come together to cultivate their own fruits, vegetables, and herbs, providing a sustainable solution to the lack of fresh produce. The garden not only improves access to nutritious foods but also fosters a sense of community and provides an educational platform for individuals to learn about gardening, nutrition, and healthy cooking.

As a result of the community garden, residents have access to a wider variety of fresh produce, enabling them to make healthier dietary choices. This leads to weight loss, improved blood sugar control, and lower rates of chronic diseases within the community. The garden becomes a source of pride and empowerment for the residents, and it serves as an example for neighboring communities to address similar challenges.

Further Reading

1. Block, D., Kouba, J. (2006). A comparison of the availability and affordability of a market basket in two communities in the Chicago area. Public Health Nutrition, 9(7), 837–845.

2. Leete, L., Bania, N., Sparks, A. (2012). Fresh Food, Fresh Advocates: Chicago's Community Health Ambassadors. Journal of Urban Health, 89(2), 177–184.

3. Loescher, L. J., Coffin, D. L., Turner, L. W. (2018). Effects of community gardens on fruit and vegetable access and intake in local communities: A systematic review. Environmental Health Perspectives, 126(11), 11001.

4. Walker, R. E., Keane, C. R., Burke, J. G. (2010). Disparities and access to healthy food in the United States: A review of food deserts literature. Health & Place, 16(5), 876–884.

Key Takeaways

- Lack of fresh produce and vitamins is a significant issue in food deserts, leading to nutrient deficiencies and poor health outcomes. - Fresh fruits and vegetables are essential sources of vitamins, minerals, and fiber, necessary for overall health and the prevention of chronic diseases. - Addressing the lack of fresh produce and vitamins requires a multifaceted approach including improving transportation options, expanding farmer's markets, promoting urban farming and community gardens, providing financial incentives, and implementing nutrition education programs. - By addressing this issue, we can improve the health and well-being of individuals living in food deserts and reduce health disparities.

Obesity trends in food deserts

Obesity is a growing public health concern globally, and its prevalence is particularly high in food deserts. In this section, we will explore the relationship between food deserts and obesity, including the contributing factors and potential solutions.

Understanding Obesity

First, let's begin by defining obesity and understanding its implications. Obesity is a condition characterized by excessive body fat accumulation, leading to negative health outcomes. Body mass index (BMI), calculated using an individual's weight and height, is commonly used to determine obesity levels. A BMI of 30 or higher is considered obese.

Obesity is a complex issue influenced by various factors, including genetics, lifestyle choices, and socio-environmental factors. It is associated with a higher risk of chronic conditions such as type 2 diabetes, heart disease, and certain cancers. Understanding the factors contributing to obesity is crucial in addressing this public health crisis.

The Relationship between Food Deserts and Obesity

Food deserts play a significant role in the development of obesity. A food desert is an area with limited access to affordable and nutritious food, typically characterized by the absence of grocery stores and an abundance of fast food outlets.

One of the main reasons for the high obesity rates in food deserts is the limited availability of fresh and healthy food options. Instead, residents often rely on unhealthy, processed, and calorie-dense foods. These food options are typically low in nutrients and high in saturated fats, added sugars, and sodium, contributing to weight gain and the prevalence of obesity.

The lack of nutritious food options is exacerbated by the abundance of fast-food restaurants and convenience stores offering energy-dense, low-quality food. These establishments often offer highly processed foods with limited nutritional value, contributing to the development of obesity.

Additionally, the socioeconomic factors associated with food deserts, such as poverty and limited access to transportation, further contribute to the obesity disparity. Low-income individuals living in food deserts may face financial constraints that limit their ability to buy and prepare healthier meals. The reliance on transportation options that are often limited in food deserts makes it challenging to access grocery stores with fresh produce and healthier food options.

Solutions to Address Obesity in Food Deserts

Addressing obesity in food deserts requires a multi-faceted approach that tackles both the lack of healthy food options and the socioeconomic factors associated with food disparities. Here are some potential solutions:

1. Increasing Access to Healthy Food: One approach is to implement policies that incentivize the establishment of grocery stores in food deserts and provide subsidies for fresh produce. This can include tax benefits, grants, and zoning regulations to promote the availability of nutritious food options.

2. Community Gardens and Urban Farming: Encouraging community gardens and urban farming initiatives can provide residents with opportunities to grow their own fresh produce. This empowers individuals to take control of their food choices, leading to improved nutrition and reduced obesity rates.

3. Nutrition Education: Implementing nutrition education programs in schools and communities can equip individuals in food deserts with knowledge and skills to make healthier food choices. These programs can focus on topics such as meal planning, cooking skills, and the benefits of a balanced diet.

4. Public Transportation and Mobile Food Markets: Improving public transportation options in food deserts can enhance access to grocery stores and farmers markets. Additionally, mobile food markets that bring fresh produce and healthier food options directly to these communities can be an effective solution.

5. Collaborative Efforts: Collaboration between local governments, community organizations, and businesses is crucial in addressing obesity in food deserts. By working together, these stakeholders can develop sustainable initiatives and interventions tailored to the specific needs of the community.

It is important to note that addressing obesity in food deserts requires a comprehensive and long-term approach. By combining these solutions and considering the unique challenges faced by each community, we can begin to combat the obesity epidemic and promote healthier lifestyles for all residents.

Summary

In this section, we explored the relationship between food deserts and obesity. We discussed how the limited availability of healthy food options and the presence of calorie-dense, low-nutrient foods contribute to obesity in these areas. Additionally, we highlighted potential solutions to address obesity in food deserts, including increasing access to healthy food, promoting community gardens, implementing nutrition education programs, improving transportation options, and fostering collaboration among stakeholders. The fight against obesity in food deserts requires a comprehensive and collaborative approach that takes into account the unique needs and challenges of these communities. By doing so, we can work towards reducing obesity rates and improving the overall health and well-being of individuals living in food deserts.

Chronic diseases associated with poor nutrition

Poor nutrition, often found in food deserts, is strongly linked to the development of chronic diseases. Chronic diseases refer to long-term health conditions that typically progress slowly and have a prolonged duration. They include conditions such as obesity, cardiovascular diseases, type 2 diabetes, and certain types of cancer. In this section, we will explore the connection between poor nutrition and these chronic diseases, highlighting the underlying mechanisms and providing examples of real-world scenarios.

Obesity as a consequence of poor nutrition

One of the most well-known chronic diseases associated with poor nutrition is obesity. Obesity is a condition characterized by an excess accumulation of body fat, often resulting from an energy imbalance between calories consumed and calories expended. In food deserts, where access to healthy and nutritious food is limited, individuals often rely on cheap and readily available processed foods that are high in calories, unhealthy fats, added sugars, and sodium.

The relationship between poor nutrition and obesity can be attributed to several factors. Firstly, the lack of affordable fresh fruits and vegetables in food deserts leads to decreased consumption of nutrient-rich foods and a higher intake of energy-dense, nutrient-poor foods. These unhealthy food choices contribute to weight gain and increased adiposity.

Additionally, poor nutrition can disrupt the regulation of appetite and satiety. Consuming foods that are high in added sugars and unhealthy fats can lead to imbalances in hormone levels, such as insulin and leptin, which play crucial roles in appetite control. This disruption can result in overeating and a higher body mass index (BMI).

Real-world example: In a study conducted in a food desert neighborhood, it was found that individuals had limited access to fresh produce and relied heavily on fast food and convenience stores for their meals. This dietary pattern, coupled with a sedentary lifestyle, resulted in a higher prevalence of obesity among the residents compared to individuals in areas with better food access.

Cardiovascular diseases and poor nutrition

Another chronic disease strongly associated with poor nutrition is cardiovascular disease (CVD). CVD encompasses a group of conditions that affect the heart and blood vessels, including coronary artery disease, heart attacks, and strokes. Poor nutrition, particularly an unhealthy diet high in saturated fats, trans fats, cholesterol, and sodium, significantly contributes to the development of CVD.

High intake of saturated and trans fats, commonly found in processed foods like fried foods, pastries, and packaged snacks, can lead to an increase in LDL cholesterol (often referred to as "bad" cholesterol) levels. When LDL cholesterol accumulates in the arteries, it can form plaque and reduce blood flow to the heart and other organs, increasing the risk of heart disease and stroke.

Excessive sodium intake, often prevalent in processed foods, can also raise blood pressure levels. High blood pressure, or hypertension, is a major risk factor for CVD, as it strains the heart and damages the blood vessels.

Real-world example: A study conducted in urban food deserts found that the residents had limited access to fresh, healthy foods and instead relied heavily on processed foods high in saturated fats and sodium. The prevalence of hypertension and heart disease was significantly higher in this population compared to individuals with better access to nutritious foods.

Type 2 diabetes and poor nutrition

Type 2 diabetes is a chronic metabolic disorder characterized by high blood glucose levels resulting from insulin resistance or insufficient insulin production. Poor nutrition, specifically a diet high in refined carbohydrates, added sugars, and unhealthy fats, is a major contributor to the development of type 2 diabetes.

Consuming a diet rich in refined carbohydrates, such as white bread, pasta, and sweetened beverages, can rapidly increase blood glucose levels. Over time, this repeated elevation of blood glucose can lead to insulin resistance, where cells become less responsive to the effects of insulin. Insulin resistance is a key component of type 2 diabetes.

Furthermore, diets high in added sugars and unhealthy fats contribute to obesity, which is a significant risk factor for type 2 diabetes. Excess body weight and adiposity can disrupt insulin signaling and lead to insulin resistance.

Real-world example: Research conducted in food desert communities found that individuals had limited access to affordable whole grains, fruits, and vegetables, and instead consumed diets high in refined carbohydrates and sugary beverages. The prevalence of type 2 diabetes in these communities was significantly higher compared to areas with better food access.

Cancer and links to poor nutrition

Poor nutrition has been recognized as a contributing factor to the development of certain types of cancer. Although diet alone may not directly cause cancer, an unhealthy diet can increase the risk of cancer development and progression.

A diet high in processed and fast foods, which are often low in fiber and high in unhealthy fats, has been linked to an increased risk of colorectal cancer. Consumption of foods high in preservatives, additives, and artificial ingredients may also contribute to carcinogenesis.

Moreover, inadequate intake of fruits and vegetables, which are rich in antioxidants and phytochemicals, can compromise the body's ability to neutralize free radicals and protect against cellular damage. This can increase the risk of various types of cancer, including lung, breast, and prostate cancer.

Real-world example: A study examining dietary patterns in a food desert area found that individuals had limited access to fresh produce and instead consumed diets high in processed and fast foods. The incidence of colorectal cancer in this population was higher compared to areas with better food access and a higher intake of fruits and vegetables.

In conclusion, poor nutrition in food deserts contributes significantly to the development of chronic diseases such as obesity, cardiovascular diseases, type 2 diabetes, and certain types of cancer. The lack of access to affordable and healthy food options leads to an increased consumption of calorie-dense, nutrient-poor foods, setting the stage for these chronic diseases. Addressing the issue of food deserts and promoting access to nutritious foods is crucial in preventing and reducing the burden of these chronic diseases in affected communities.

Exercises:

1. Research and analyze the nutritional profiles of commonly consumed foods in your local food desert area. Identify how these foods contribute to the development of chronic diseases.

2. Design a health promotion campaign targeting individuals living in food deserts, focusing on the importance of nutrition in preventing chronic diseases. Consider creative strategies to deliver the message effectively.

Resources:

1. Drewnowski, A., & Darmon, N. (2005). Food choices and diet costs: an economic analysis. The Journal of nutrition, 135(4), 900–904. 2. Mozaffarian, D., & Rimm, E. B. (2010). The interaction between nutrition and infection. Clinical Infectious Diseases, 46(10), 1582–1588. 3. World Cancer Research Fund/American Institute for Cancer Research. Diet, Nutrition, Physical Activity and Cancer: A Global Perspective. Continuous Update Project Expert Report 2018. 4. American Heart Association. (2021). Diet and Lifestyle Recommendations. Retrieved from https://www.heart.org/en/healthy-living/healthy-eating/eat-smart/nutrition-basics/diet-a

Tricks and Caveats:

1. It is important to acknowledge that chronic diseases have multifactorial causes, and poor nutrition is just one aspect. It is crucial to consider other factors such as genetic predisposition, lifestyle factors, and environmental influences in the development of chronic diseases.

2. Avoid generalizing all processed foods as unhealthy. Some processed foods can be part of a balanced diet if they are low in added sugars, sodium, and unhealthy fats. Read food labels and choose processed foods wisely.

Unconventional Approach:

Utilize innovative technology such as mobile applications that provide personalized nutrition recommendations and grocery lists based on an individual's health status and the availability of local food options in food deserts. These apps can help bridge the gap between poor nutrition and chronic diseases by empowering individuals with the knowledge and resources to make healthier food choices within their limited food environment.

Mental Health and Food Deserts

Psychological effects of food insecurity

Food insecurity, which refers to a lack of consistent access to nutritious and culturally appropriate food, has profound psychological effects on individuals and communities. The experience of food insecurity can lead to a range of emotional and mental health challenges, contributing to increased stress, anxiety, depression, and a decreased sense of well-being.

One of the primary psychological effects of food insecurity is the development of chronic stress. When individuals are uncertain about where their next meal will come from or if they will have enough food to feed themselves and their families, it creates a constant state of heightened stress and worry. This chronic stress can disrupt normal physiological and psychological functioning, leading to a variety of negative outcomes.

In addition to the immediate stress response, food insecurity can also contribute to increased levels of anxiety. The uncertainty and unpredictability associated with not having enough food can lead to feelings of unease, fear, and a constant sense of heightened vigilance. Those experiencing food insecurity may constantly worry about whether they will have enough food to meet their basic needs, leading to chronic and debilitating anxiety.

The psychological effects of food insecurity extend beyond stress and anxiety and can also contribute to the development or exacerbation of mental health disorders such as depression. The experience of not having enough food can lead to feelings of sadness, hopelessness, and a loss of motivation. Moreover, the lack of proper nutrition associated with food insecurity can contribute to imbalances in brain chemistry and neurotransmitter function, which are known to play a role in the development of depression.

Food insecurity can also have significant implications for self-esteem and overall psychological well-being. When individuals are unable to consistently provide nutritious food for themselves and their families, they may feel a sense of shame, guilt, or failure. This can lead to a negative self-perception and a diminished sense of self-worth, impacting their overall psychological well-being and quality of life.

For children, the psychological effects of food insecurity can be particularly detrimental. Inadequate access to nutritious food during critical periods of brain development can lead to long-term cognitive and behavioral challenges. Children who experience food insecurity may have difficulty concentrating in school, exhibit behavioral problems, and experience delays in physical and emotional development.

Addressing the psychological effects of food insecurity requires a comprehensive approach that goes beyond simply providing access to food. It involves addressing the underlying causes of food insecurity, such as poverty, lack of employment opportunities, and systemic inequities. It also requires integrating mental health support and resources into food assistance programs and ensuring that individuals and communities have access to culturally appropriate and affordable mental health services.

One example of an intervention that addresses the psychological effects of food insecurity is the implementation of trauma-informed care within food assistance programs. Trauma-informed care recognizes the potential trauma and stress associated with the experience of food insecurity and provides support and resources to individuals in a sensitive and compassionate manner. This approach acknowledges the impact of food insecurity on mental health and seeks to create a safe and supportive environment for individuals to access nutritious food and mental health services.

In conclusion, food insecurity has significant psychological effects on individuals and communities. It contributes to chronic stress, anxiety, depression, and a diminished sense of self-worth. Addressing the psychological effects of food insecurity requires a holistic approach that integrates mental health support and resources into food assistance programs, addresses the underlying causes of food insecurity, and promotes systemic change to create a more equitable and just food system.

Food Deserts and Mental Health Disorders

Food deserts, characterized by limited access to affordable and nutritious food options, have been associated with various health issues, including mental health disorders. The lack of access to fresh, healthy foods in food deserts can have a detrimental impact on psychological well-being. In this section, we will explore the relationship between food deserts and mental health disorders, examining the mechanisms through which food insecurity can contribute to mental health problems and discussing potential strategies to address this issue.

The Link between Food Insecurity and Mental Health

Food insecurity, a common consequence of living in a food desert, refers to the limited or uncertain availability of nutritionally adequate and safe foods. This uncertainty and lack of access to sufficient food can lead to chronic stress, anxiety, and depression, which are known risk factors for the development of mental health disorders. Studies have consistently shown a higher prevalence of mental health disorders, such as depression and anxiety, among individuals living in food deserts compared to those with adequate access to healthy food options.

One proposed mechanism linking food insecurity and mental health disorders is the physiological impact of nutrient deficiencies. In food deserts, where fresh fruits, vegetables, and other nutrient-rich foods are scarce, individuals may rely on cheaper and easily accessible processed foods that are often high in sugar, unhealthy fats, and low in essential nutrients. Insufficient intake of key vitamins and minerals, such as omega-3 fatty acids, B vitamins, and iron, can disrupt neurotransmitter production and brain function, contributing to mood disorders.

Additionally, stress plays a significant role in the relationship between food deserts and mental health disorders. Living in a food desert often entails dealing with socio-economic challenges, financial constraints, and food-related stress, all of which can contribute to chronic stress. The constant worry and uncertainty about food availability can heighten stress levels, leading to mental health problems.

Addressing Mental Health Concerns in Food Deserts

Recognizing the impact of food deserts on mental health is crucial for developing interventions and strategies to address this issue. Here, we discuss a multifaceted approach to mitigate mental health problems associated with food deserts:

1. **Improve access to nutritious foods:** A key intervention is to increase the availability and affordability of healthy food options in food deserts. This can be achieved through initiatives such as establishing community gardens, supporting local farmers markets, and incentivizing grocery stores to open in underserved areas.

2. **Nutrition education and mental health promotion:** Providing nutrition education and mental health promotion programs to individuals living in food deserts can empower them to make informed food choices and manage their mental well-being effectively. Educational programs can focus on the importance of a balanced diet, the relationship between nutrition and mental health, and stress management techniques.

3. **Mental health support services:** Access to mental health support services, including counseling and therapy, should be made readily available for individuals living in food deserts. Collaborations between community organizations, healthcare providers, and mental health professionals can facilitate the provision of affordable and accessible mental health care.

4. **Social support and community engagement:** Building a sense of community and fostering social support networks can help alleviate the mental health burden in food deserts. Community organizations and grassroots initiatives can organize activities that promote social interaction, such as community meals, support groups, and neighborhood events.

5. **Policy changes:** Advocacy for policy changes at the local, state, and national levels can play a critical role in addressing mental health concerns in food deserts. Policies that promote food security, equitable access to healthy foods, and mental health support can contribute to long-term improvements in individual and community mental well-being.

Case Study: Farm-to-School Programs

One successful intervention that addresses both nutrition and mental health concerns in food deserts is the implementation of farm-to-school programs. These programs facilitate the procurement of locally grown, fresh produce for schools in food desert areas. By incorporating these nutritious foods into school meals, farm-to-school programs not only improve children's access to healthy foods but also promote education around nutrition and mental well-being.

Farm-to-school programs also provide opportunities for students to engage in hands-on activities related to food production, such as gardening and cooking workshops. These activities foster a sense of connection to the food system, promote a positive food environment, and contribute to positive mental health outcomes. Furthermore, farm-to-school programs stimulate the local economy by supporting local farmers and creating sustainable food systems.

Conclusion

The relationship between food deserts and mental health disorders is a significant public health concern. Food insecurity, limited access to nutritious foods, and chronic stress associated with living in food deserts can contribute to the development and exacerbation of mental health problems. Addressing this issue requires a comprehensive approach that includes improving access to healthy foods, providing nutrition education, enhancing mental health support services, fostering community engagement, and advocating for policy changes. By implementing these strategies, we can help mitigate the negative impact of food deserts on mental health and promote overall well-being in affected populations.

Addressing mental health concerns in food deserts

Food deserts are not just a matter of physical access to healthy food options; they also have significant implications for mental health. Limited access to nutritious food can lead to a range of psychological effects, including increased stress, anxiety, and depression. In this section, we will explore the various ways in which mental health concerns can be addressed in the context of food deserts.

Understanding the Psychological Effects of Food Insecurity

Food insecurity, which is a common characteristic of food deserts, refers to the lack of consistent access to enough nutritious food for an active and healthy lifestyle. This chronic condition is known to have adverse effects on mental health. It can lead to feelings of deprivation, uncertainty, and chronic stress, which can significantly impact an individual's overall well-being.

Research has shown that individuals living in food deserts are more likely to experience symptoms of anxiety and depression compared to those with better access to healthy food options. The constant struggle to find affordable and nutritious food can create a sense of hopelessness and helplessness, which can further exacerbate mental health issues.

Moreover, the reliance on cheaper, processed, and high-sugar foods commonly found in food deserts can negatively impact brain function and mood regulation. Nutritional deficiencies, particularly a lack of essential vitamins and minerals, can contribute to mood disorders and cognitive impairments.

Promoting Mental Health in Food Deserts

Addressing mental health concerns in food deserts requires a comprehensive approach that focuses on both individual and community-level interventions. Here are some strategies that can be implemented:

1. **Increase access to mental health services:** One of the key steps in addressing mental health concerns in food deserts is to improve access to mental health services. This could involve partnering with local healthcare providers, community-based organizations, and mental health professionals to establish mobile clinics or satellite centers in underserved areas. These facilities can provide mental health screenings, counseling, therapy, and psychiatric support.

2. **Implement community-based support networks:** Creating community-based support networks can help individuals in food deserts feel more connected and supported. These networks can facilitate group therapy sessions, peer support groups, and workshops on mental health literacy and coping strategies. It is essential to engage community members and empower them to take an active role in addressing mental health concerns.

3. **Promote mental health education and awareness:** Implementing mental health education programs in schools, community centers, and local organizations can significantly contribute to raising awareness and reducing the stigma associated with seeking help for mental health issues. These programs can focus on enhancing mental health literacy, providing coping skills, and promoting self-care practices.

4. **Encourage physical activity and social engagement:** Physical activity has been shown to have a positive impact on mental health. Creating safe spaces for exercise and recreational activities within food deserts can help improve mental well-being. Additionally, promoting social engagement through community events, sports activities, and volunteer programs can foster a sense of belonging and social support.

5. **Collaborate with local food assistance programs:** Collaborating with local food assistance programs, such as food banks and pantries, can help ensure that individuals in food deserts have access to a more diverse range of nutritious food options. These partnerships can also include mental health screenings and referrals to support services within the food assistance programs.

Case Study: The Fresh Food Pharmacy

The Fresh Food Pharmacy program, developed by Geisinger Health System in Pennsylvania, is an example of an innovative approach to address mental health concerns in food deserts. This program combines access to nutritious food with comprehensive healthcare services.

Participants in the program receive tailored meal plans that prioritize fresh fruits, vegetables, lean proteins, and whole grains. They also receive ongoing support from a multidisciplinary team of healthcare professionals, including registered dietitians, pharmacists, and behavioral health specialists.

The program aims to improve mental health outcomes by providing individuals with the necessary resources to improve their diet and overall well-being. By addressing both the physical and mental aspects of health, the Fresh Food Pharmacy program has demonstrated promising results in improving mental health outcomes and overall quality of life for participants.

Conclusion

Addressing mental health concerns in food deserts is a crucial aspect of improving overall well-being and reducing health disparities. By implementing strategies that focus on increasing access to mental health services, promoting mental health education, and fostering community support networks, we can empower individuals in food deserts to take control of their mental well-being.

It is important to recognize that mental health interventions in food deserts should be culturally sensitive and tailored to the specific needs of the community. By adopting a holistic approach that integrates physical health, mental health, and community engagement, we can make significant strides in addressing mental health concerns and building healthier and more resilient communities in food deserts.

Childhood Development and Food Deserts

Early childhood nutrition and brain development

Early childhood is a critical period for brain development, and proper nutrition plays a key role in ensuring optimal growth and cognitive function. During this stage, the brain undergoes rapid development, and the nutrients children receive from their diet are essential for supporting this process. In this section, we will explore the importance of early childhood nutrition for brain development, the specific nutrients that are crucial during this period, and the long-term consequences of inadequate nutrition.

Importance of early childhood nutrition

The early years of life are a period of rapid brain growth and development. The brain develops most rapidly during the first three years of life, with connections between brain cells, known as synapses, forming at a remarkable pace. Proper nutrition is crucial during this period as it provides the building blocks for brain development and helps establish a strong foundation for cognitive, emotional, and physical health.

Key nutrients for brain development

Several nutrients play a critical role in supporting brain development in early childhood. These include:

1. Omega-3 fatty acids: Omega-3 fatty acids, especially docosahexaenoic acid (DHA), are essential for brain development and function. DHA makes up a significant portion of the brain's cell membranes and is involved in various processes, including neural signaling and inflammation regulation. Good sources of omega-3 fatty acids include fatty fish (such as salmon and sardines), chia seeds, flaxseeds, and walnuts.

2. Iron: Iron is essential for the production of hemoglobin, the protein that carries oxygen to the brain and other organs. Iron deficiency in early childhood can lead to cognitive impairments and behavioral problems. Good sources of iron include lean meats, eggs, legumes, and fortified cereals.

3. Iodine: Iodine is necessary for the production of thyroid hormones, which are crucial for brain development and function. Inadequate iodine intake during pregnancy and early childhood can lead to cognitive impairments, including intellectual disabilities. Good sources of iodine include iodized salt, seafood, and dairy products.

4. Vitamin B12: Vitamin B12 is involved in the production of myelin, the protective covering of nerve fibers. Adequate intake of vitamin B12 during early childhood is crucial for proper brain development and function. Good sources of vitamin B12 include animal products such as meat, fish, eggs, and dairy.

5. Choline: Choline is essential for the synthesis of acetylcholine, a neurotransmitter involved in memory and learning. Adequate choline intake during early childhood supports brain development and cognitive function. Good sources of choline include eggs, liver, fish, and soybeans.

These are just a few examples of the many nutrients that are important for brain development. A balanced diet that includes a variety of nutrient-rich foods is key to providing young children with the necessary nutrients for optimal brain growth.

Consequences of inadequate nutrition

Inadequate nutrition during early childhood can have long-term consequences on brain development and overall health. Here are some of the potential impacts:

1. Cognitive impairments: Poor nutrition in early childhood can lead to cognitive impairments, including lower IQ, learning difficulties, and reduced academic achievement. Inadequate intake of key nutrients such as omega-3 fatty acids, iron, and iodine can impair neural development and compromise cognitive function.

2. Behavioral problems: Children who experience inadequate nutrition in early childhood are at a higher risk of developing behavioral problems, including attention-deficit/hyperactivity disorder (ADHD) and conduct disorders. Nutrient deficiencies can disrupt neurochemical processes and affect brain regions involved in behavior regulation.

3. Increased risk of mental health disorders: Inadequate nutrition during early childhood has been linked to an increased risk of mental health disorders later in life, including depression, anxiety, and schizophrenia. Proper

nutrition is important for the development and functioning of neurotransmitters and other biochemical processes that influence mental health.

4. Impaired physical growth: Inadequate nutrition can also result in stunted physical growth, including poor weight gain and shorter stature. Proper nutrition supports overall growth and development, including the growth of the brain and other organs.

It is important to note that the effects of early childhood nutrition on brain development are not solely determined by the availability of nutrients, but also by environmental factors such as stimulation and nurturing caregiving. Adequate nutrition, coupled with a supportive and stimulating environment, provides the best opportunity for optimal brain development and overall well-being.

Promoting early childhood nutrition

Ensuring proper nutrition during early childhood is essential for supporting optimal brain development. Here are some strategies to promote early childhood nutrition:

1. Education and awareness: Providing parents, caregivers, and healthcare professionals with information about the importance of early childhood nutrition and the specific nutrients needed for brain development can help promote healthy eating habits.

2. Access to nutritious foods: Enhancing access to affordable, nutrient-rich foods in communities, particularly in areas with limited food options, can play a crucial role in improving early childhood nutrition. This can involve initiatives such as farmers markets, community gardens, and programs that provide healthy meals in early childhood settings.

3. Early intervention: Identifying and addressing nutritional deficiencies and inadequate diets early on can prevent long-term detrimental effects on brain development. Regular screenings and assessments can help identify children at risk and ensure appropriate interventions.

4. Parental and caregiver education: Providing parents and caregivers with the knowledge and skills to make informed decisions about nutrition and feeding practices can empower them to provide optimal nutrition for their children. This can include information on age-appropriate foods, portion sizes, and strategies to encourage healthy eating habits.

5. Collaboration and policy support: Collaboration between various stakeholders, including healthcare professionals, policymakers, educators, and community organizations, is essential in creating comprehensive strategies to promote early childhood nutrition. Supportive policies, such as nutritional standards for childcare settings and schools, can also help create an environment conducive to healthy eating habits.

By prioritizing early childhood nutrition and implementing multifaceted strategies, we can help promote the healthy development of young children's brains and set them on a path towards a brighter future.

Conclusion

Proper nutrition during early childhood is crucial for optimal brain development. Nutrients such as omega-3 fatty acids, iron, iodine, vitamin B12, and choline play essential roles in supporting brain growth and function. Inadequate nutrition during this critical period can have long-term consequences, including cognitive impairments, behavioral problems, and increased risk of mental health disorders. Promoting early childhood nutrition requires education, access to healthy foods, early intervention, parental and caregiver support, and collaboration among various stakeholders. By investing in early childhood nutrition, we can give children the best possible start in life and support their overall well-being and success.

Academic Performance and Food Access

Academic performance and food access are interconnected in complex ways. Adequate nutrition is crucial for cognitive development, learning, and overall academic achievement. However, in food deserts where nutritious food options are limited, students may face challenges that hinder their educational outcomes. This section explores the relationship between academic performance and food access, highlighting the impact of food deserts on students and discussing potential strategies to mitigate the negative effects.

The Importance of Nutrition for Academic Performance

Nutrition plays a vital role in the cognitive development and functioning of individuals, especially during childhood and adolescence. Adequate intake of essential nutrients such as vitamins, minerals, and omega-3 fatty acids is essential for brain development and functioning. These nutrients support various cognitive processes, including attention span, memory retention, and problem-solving skills.

Multiple studies have shown a positive correlation between good nutrition and academic performance. For example, a study conducted by Rampersaud et al. (2005) found that students who consumed a healthy breakfast had improved cognitive function, attention, memory, and academic performance compared to those who skipped breakfast or consumed an unhealthy meal. Similarly, Jansen et al. (2014) demonstrated that a well-balanced diet, rich in fruits, vegetables, whole grains, and lean proteins, was associated with higher academic achievement.

Challenges Faced by Students in Food Deserts

Students living in food deserts face unique challenges that can negatively impact their academic performance. Food deserts are characterized by limited access to affordable and nutritious food, often resulting in a higher consumption of unhealthy processed foods and a lack of fresh produce. Consequently, students in food deserts may experience nutritional deficiencies, including inadequate intake of essential vitamins, minerals, and other nutrients crucial for brain development and function.

These nutritional deficiencies can have a direct impact on students' cognitive abilities, attention span, and memory retention, making it difficult for them to concentrate and learn effectively. Furthermore, food deserts are often associated with higher levels of food insecurity, leading to irregular eating patterns and hunger, which can further impede students' ability to focus and participate actively in academic activities.

Strategies to Improve Food Access and Academic Performance

Addressing the challenges faced by students in food deserts requires multifaceted interventions that focus on improving food access and promoting healthy eating habits. Here are some strategies that can help enhance academic performance by ensuring adequate nutrition:

School-based Nutritional Programs Schools play a crucial role in promoting healthy eating habits and improving food access for students. Implementing school-based nutritional programs, such as providing free or reduced-price breakfast and lunch, can ensure that students receive at least two nutritious meals during the day. These programs should prioritize offering a variety of fruits, vegetables, whole grains, and lean proteins to meet students' nutritional needs.

Community Gardens and Farm-to-School Programs Community gardens and farm-to-school programs can play a significant role in addressing food deserts by providing fresh and locally grown produce to schools. These initiatives enable students to learn about agriculture, nutrition, and food production while increasing access to fresh and nutritious food. Additionally, involving students in these programs can empower them to make healthier food choices and develop a positive relationship with food.

Nutrition Education and Cooking Classes Integrating nutrition education and cooking classes into the curriculum can help students develop essential knowledge and skills related to healthy eating. These classes can teach students about the benefits of a balanced diet, how to prepare nutritious meals on a budget, and the importance of making informed food choices. Empowering students with nutrition knowledge can positively influence their food preferences and contribute to improved academic performance.

Partnerships with Local Food Retailers Collaborating with local food retailers, such as grocery stores and farmers markets, can increase access to affordable and nutritious food for students in food deserts. Schools can establish partnerships to provide transportation or organize regular visits to these retailers, ensuring that students have access to a wide range of fresh and healthy food options. These partnerships can also promote community engagement and support local businesses.

Case Study: The Food Education Empowerment and Sustainability Team (FEEST)

The Food Education Empowerment and Sustainability Team (FEEST) is a community-based organization operating in Seattle, Washington. FEEST works with high school students from diverse backgrounds to address food justice and improve their access to healthy food options. The organization focuses on empowering students to advocate for changes in school food policies and creating a supportive environment for healthy eating.

FEEST's approach involves various strategies to enhance food access and improve academic performance. They organize cooking workshops, where students learn to prepare nutritious meals using locally sourced ingredients. These workshops not only teach essential cooking skills but also provide an opportunity for students to understand the importance of a healthy diet and its impact on academic performance.

Furthermore, FEEST collaborates with local farmers markets and community gardens to increase the availability of fresh produce in schools. By connecting students directly with local food sources, FEEST aims to foster a sense of ownership and appreciation for healthy food choices.

Preliminary evaluations of FEEST's programs have shown promising results. Students involved in FEEST reported an improved understanding of nutrition and an increased consumption of fruits and vegetables. Additionally, participants demonstrated a stronger sense of agency and advocacy skills, leading to successful grassroots campaigns for healthier food options within their schools.

Conclusion

Access to nutritious food is a fundamental requirement for academic success. Students in food deserts face significant challenges due to limited access to affordable and nutritious food options, which can have negative implications for their cognitive development and academic performance. However, through targeted interventions such as school-based nutritional programs, community partnerships, and nutrition education initiatives, it is possible to improve food access and positively impact students' academic outcomes.

Ensuring that all students have access to healthy and nutritious meals is not only an educational imperative but also a matter of social justice. By addressing food deserts and promoting healthy eating habits, we can create a supportive environment that enables students to thrive academically and reach their full potential. It is essential for policymakers, educators, and communities to work together in implementing comprehensive strategies that prioritize nutrition and academic success for all students.

Long-term consequences of food deserts on children

Food deserts, characterized by limited access to affordable and nutritious food, have profound effects on the health and well-being of children. The long-term consequences of growing up in food deserts can have lasting impacts on their physical and cognitive development, academic performance, and overall quality of life. In this section, we will explore these consequences in detail and discuss potential solutions to mitigate their effects.

Physical Health Effects

One of the most immediate and significant consequences of food deserts for children is the increased risk of poor physical health. Limited access to fresh fruits, vegetables, and other nutritious foods can lead to a higher consumption of processed and unhealthy foods. This diet lacking in essential nutrients, vitamins, and minerals can result in malnutrition and a higher prevalence of conditions such as obesity, type 2 diabetes, and cardiovascular diseases.

Children who grow up in food deserts often face challenges in maintaining a healthy weight. The lack of access to fresh produce and healthier food options promotes the consumption of calorie-dense, nutrient-poor foods. As a result, children may develop unhealthy eating habits and struggle with weight management, increasing the risk of obesity and related health problems. Obesity, in turn, contributes to a variety of health issues including high blood pressure, joint problems, and sleep disorders.

Cognitive Development and Academic Performance

The impact of food deserts on children goes beyond physical health. Inadequate nutrition can also impair cognitive development and academic performance. Proper nutrition, especially during early childhood, is crucial for optimal brain growth and function. Essential nutrients such as omega-3 fatty acids, iron, and B vitamins play a vital role in the development of cognitive skills, memory, attention, and problem-solving abilities.

Children who lack access to nutritious food may experience difficulties in concentration, memory, and processing information. They may exhibit lower academic achievement and struggle with cognitive tasks requiring critical thinking and problem-solving skills. The consequences of poor nutrition on cognitive development can have long-lasting effects, affecting a child's educational attainment and future opportunities.

Emotional and Behavioral Effects

Living in food deserts can also take a toll on children's emotional and behavioral well-being. Food insecurity and limited access to nutritious food can cause chronic stress and anxiety. Stressors related to food scarcity can disrupt healthy emotional regulation in children and increase the risk of mental health issues such as depression, anxiety disorders, and other behavioral problems.

Furthermore, inadequate nutrition can affect the production of neurotransmitters in the brain, including serotonin and dopamine, which are crucial for regulating mood and emotions. Imbalances in these neurotransmitters due to poor nutrition can lead to mood disorders, behavioral issues, and difficulty in managing emotions.

Food Deserts and Generational Cycle of Health Inequity

The long-term consequences of food deserts on children are not limited to their individual health outcomes. There is a risk of perpetuating a generational cycle of health inequity. Children growing up in food deserts may adopt unhealthy habits and attitudes towards food, passing them on to their own children in the future.

Inadequate nutrition and health problems can have intergenerational effects, impacting the health outcomes of future generations. Breaking this cycle requires addressing not only the physical access to nutritious food but also the educational, economic, and social factors that contribute to food deserts.

Addressing the Long-term Consequences

Mitigating the long-term consequences of food deserts on children requires a comprehensive approach that addresses the root causes of food inequity and promotes access to healthy food options. Some potential strategies include:

1. Increasing the availability of fresh and nutritious food options in food deserts through policies and initiatives that attract grocery stores and farmers markets to underserved areas. 2. Supporting community-driven solutions such as urban gardens and community-supported agriculture programs that promote local food production and distribution. 3. Implementing nutrition education programs in schools to teach children and their families about healthy eating habits and the importance of nutritious food choices. 4. Strengthening social safety nets and increasing access to affordable and nutritious food through programs such as school breakfast and lunch programs, WIC (Women, Infants, and Children) assistance, and SNAP (Supplemental Nutrition Assistance Program).

It is important to approach these interventions from an equity and social justice perspective, ensuring that everyone, regardless of their socioeconomic background, has access to nutritious food options. Addressing the long-term consequences of food deserts on children requires a multi-sectoral approach involving policymakers, community organizations, healthcare professionals, educators, and individuals working together to create sustainable and lasting solutions.

By addressing the long-term consequences of food deserts on children, we can improve their overall health and well-being, break the generational cycle of health inequity, and create a future where every child has equal access to nutritious food and the opportunity to thrive.

Food Deserts and Environmental Health

Environmental Pollution and Food Deserts

Environmental pollution plays a significant role in exacerbating the challenges faced by food deserts. Polluted environments not only limit the availability of nutritious food but also contribute to the health risks associated with living in these areas. In this section, we will explore the link between environmental pollution and food deserts, examine the impact on local ecosystems, and discuss the need for sustainable food systems and environmental justice.

Pollution and Limited Access to Healthy Food

One of the main consequences of environmental pollution in food deserts is the limited access to healthy food options. Pollution can affect the quality and availability of fresh produce, making it difficult for residents to obtain nutritious food. Heavy metals, pesticides, and other pollutants can contaminate soil, water sources, and crops, rendering them unsafe for consumption.

For example, industrial pollution in urban food deserts may lead to soil contamination, making it unsuitable for cultivating fruits and vegetables. This can result in a scarcity of fresh, locally grown produce, forcing residents to rely on processed and unhealthy food from convenience stores or fast food outlets. Areas near industrial plants or highways may also experience higher levels of air pollution, which can impact the quality and safety of food.

Health Risks Associated with Pollution in Food Deserts

The presence of pollution in food deserts poses significant health risks to the residents. Exposure to pollutants can lead to various adverse health effects, such as respiratory problems, cardiovascular diseases, and even cancer. These health risks are further exacerbated by the limited availability of nutritious food options, creating a detrimental cycle of poor health outcomes.

For instance, air pollution caused by nearby factories or heavy traffic can increase the risk of respiratory conditions like asthma. The combination of air pollution and poor nutrition in food deserts contributes to higher rates of chronic diseases, including obesity, diabetes, and hypertension. This highlights the importance of addressing both environmental pollution and limited food access to improve the overall health of individuals in food desert communities.

Impact on Local Ecosystems

The presence of food deserts can also have a significant impact on local ecosystems. The lack of access to healthy and sustainably produced food can lead to increased demand for processed and mass-produced alternatives, which have negative consequences for the environment.

For example, the reliance on fast food outlets and convenience stores in food deserts promotes the consumption of highly processed and packaged foods, contributing to increased waste generation and carbon emissions. Additionally, the lack of locally grown food encourages the transportation of produce from distant regions, leading to increased fuel consumption and greenhouse gas emissions.

Sustainable Food Systems and Environmental Justice

Addressing environmental pollution in food deserts requires the development of sustainable food systems that prioritize environmental protection and access to nutritious food. This involves promoting sustainable farming practices, reducing waste, and supporting local food production.

One approach is the implementation of urban agriculture initiatives, such as community gardens and rooftop farming. These initiatives not only provide residents with access to fresh produce but also contribute to the reduction of pollution and greenhouse gas emissions by eliminating the need for long-distance transportation.

Furthermore, promoting environmental justice is crucial in addressing the disparities faced by food desert communities. Environmental justice advocates for fair distribution of environmental benefits and burdens, ensuring that vulnerable communities are not disproportionately affected by pollution. This involves engaging with residents, advocating for policy changes, and holding polluting industries accountable for their actions.

By combining sustainable food systems and environmental justice efforts, we can work towards creating healthier and more equitable environments for individuals living in food deserts.

Summary

In this section, we explored the link between environmental pollution and food deserts. We discussed how pollution limits access to healthy food options and contributes to health risks for residents. We also highlighted the impact of food deserts on local ecosystems and the need for sustainable food systems and environmental justice. By addressing environmental pollution and promoting access to nutritious food, we can improve the overall health and well-being of individuals living in food desert communities.

Impact of food deserts on local ecosystems

Food deserts not only have profound effects on the access to nutritious food for individuals and communities, but they also have significant impacts on local ecosystems. The limited availability of healthy food options in these areas leads to various environmental consequences that affect both the natural environment and human populations.

One of the major effects of food deserts on local ecosystems is the increased reliance on processed and packaged foods. In the absence of fresh produce and healthy food choices, people living in food deserts often turn to unhealthy packaged snacks and processed foods, which are typically high in calories, unhealthy fats, and sugars. The consumption of such foods leads to increased waste generation, as most of these products come in non-recyclable packaging. Consequently, the disposal of these packaging materials contributes to landfills and pollution, further adding to the environmental burden.

The lack of fresh and locally sourced food in food deserts also means that a significant portion of the food consumed is imported from outside the local region. This long-distance transportation of food contributes to greenhouse gas emissions from the burning of fossil fuels, which in turn contributes to climate change. Additionally, the transportation of food over long distances requires the use of refrigerated trucks or planes, further increasing energy consumption and carbon emissions. These environmental impacts exacerbate the already existing challenges associated with climate change and sustainable food production.

Moreover, the absence of local food sources in food deserts means that the agricultural land in these areas is often underutilized or abandoned. This leads to a loss of biodiversity and ecological balance, as the natural habitat is disrupted and becomes vulnerable to invasive species and other environmental stressors. The decline in agricultural activity and local food production also results in the loss of traditional farming practices and knowledge, further distancing communities from their connection to the land and natural resources.

To mitigate the negative impact of food deserts on local ecosystems, several strategies can be implemented. One approach is to promote urban farming and community gardens within food desert areas. These initiatives not only provide fresh and locally grown produce but also encourage sustainable agriculture practices, reduce food waste, and enhance the environmental resilience of the community. Additionally, supporting local farmers and food producers can help stimulate the local economy and reduce the carbon footprint associated with long-distance food transportation.

Furthermore, adopting sustainable food systems and agroecological practices can contribute to the preservation of biodiversity and the restoration of degraded ecosystems. These practices prioritize the use of organic and environmentally friendly farming techniques, reducing the reliance on chemical inputs and promoting ecological balance. By fostering a closer connection between food production and ecological conservation, food deserts can become hubs for environmental stewardship and sustainability.

It is important to recognize that addressing the impact of food deserts on local ecosystems requires a multi-faceted and interdisciplinary approach. Collaboration between various stakeholders, including government agencies, community organizations, researchers, and policymakers, is crucial to develop and implement effective strategies. By acknowledging the intricate relationship between food access, environmental sustainability, and human well-being, we can work towards creating food systems that are equitable, environmentally responsible, and supportive of local ecosystems.

In conclusion, food deserts not only contribute to nutritional inequalities but also have significant impacts on local ecosystems. The reliance on processed foods and long-distance food transportation leads to increased waste generation and greenhouse gas emissions. The underutilization of agricultural land and loss of local food sources further disrupts ecosystems and biodiversity. However, by promoting sustainable farming practices, supporting local producers, and fostering community-based initiatives, we can mitigate the environmental consequences of food deserts while ensuring access to healthy and nutritious food for all.

Sustainable Food Systems and Environmental Justice

In the context of food deserts, addressing issues related to sustainable food systems and environmental justice is crucial. Sustainable food systems aim to provide nutritious food while minimizing the negative impact on the environment. Environmental justice focuses on the fair distribution of environmental benefits and burdens, including access to healthy and sustainable food options. By integrating sustainable practices and addressing environmental disparities, we can contribute to the overall well-being of communities affected by food deserts.

Understanding Sustainable Food Systems

A sustainable food system encompasses various aspects, including production, distribution, consumption, and waste management. It emphasizes the conservation of natural resources, promotes biodiversity, and minimizes pollution and waste throughout the entire food supply chain.

One of the key principles of sustainable food systems is promoting agroecology. Agroecology encourages ecological practices in agriculture, such as organic farming, crop rotation, and integrated pest management. These methods reduce the use of synthetic pesticides and fertilizers, protect soil health, and support biodiversity.

Another important aspect of sustainable food systems is reducing food waste. According to the Food and Agriculture Organization (FAO), approximately one-third of the food produced globally is lost or wasted. Implementing strategies to minimize food waste, such as better storage and transportation practices, can help increase food availability and reduce the environmental impact of food production.

Environmental Justice in Food Deserts

Environmental justice addresses the unequal distribution of environmental benefits and burdens, particularly in marginalized communities. In the context of food deserts, environmental justice focuses on ensuring equitable access to healthy and sustainable food options.

In many food desert communities, residents are disproportionately exposed to environmental hazards, such as pollution from industrial activities. These environmental burdens can exacerbate health issues and perpetuate inequalities. By promoting environmental justice, we can strive to create healthier and more sustainable living environments for everyone.

Addressing environmental justice in food deserts involves recognizing the systemic factors that contribute to inequalities. It includes understanding the historical and socio-economic context that has led to the concentration of food deserts in certain neighborhoods, often in low-income communities. By acknowledging these disparities, we can work towards implementing policies and interventions that promote equity in accessing healthy food.

Promoting Sustainable Food Systems in Food Deserts

Integrating sustainable food systems in food deserts can significantly contribute to improving access to nutritious and environmentally friendly food options. Here are some strategies and examples of initiatives that can be implemented:

1. Community Gardens and Urban Agriculture: Encouraging community-led initiatives to create gardens and urban farms can empower residents to grow their own food, increasing access to fresh produce. These initiatives not only provide nutritious food but also promote community engagement and education about sustainable agriculture.

2. Local Food Networks: Establishing local food networks can connect small-scale farmers and food producers with consumers in food desert areas. These networks can facilitate the distribution of fresh and locally grown food, reducing the reliance on long-distance transportation and supporting local economies.

3. Sustainable Food Access Programs: Collaborating with local farmers markets, food cooperatives, and community-supported agriculture (CSA) initiatives can provide sustainable food options directly to food desert communities. These programs can offer fresh produce, organic foods, and other environmentally friendly food products at affordable prices.

4. Food Recovery and Redistribution: Implementing programs to collect surplus food from restaurants, grocery stores, and farms can help minimize food waste and redistribute it to communities in need. This approach reduces environmental impact and provides nutritious food to individuals living in food deserts.

5. Education and Awareness: Educating residents of food deserts about sustainable food choices, including the importance of organic and locally sourced products, can empower individuals to make informed decisions. This education can be delivered through workshops, community programs, and school curricula.

6. Policy and Planning: Incorporating sustainable food system considerations into urban planning and policy development can help address environmental disparities in food deserts. This may involve zoning regulations that promote farmers markets or community gardens, incentivizing sustainable farming practices, and integrating food access considerations into transportation planning.

Case Study: The Philadelphia Food Justice Initiative

The Philadelphia Food Justice Initiative is an example of a comprehensive approach to addressing environmental justice and promoting sustainable food systems in food deserts. This initiative aims to increase access to healthy food, support local economies, and improve the overall food environment in Philadelphia.

One of the key strategies of the initiative is the implementation of the Philadelphia Land Bank. This program converts vacant and underutilized land into opportunities for urban agriculture and community gardening. Through the Land Bank, community organizations and individuals can transform vacant lots into productive spaces, providing fresh produce and educational opportunities to residents.

Additionally, the Philadelphia Food Justice Initiative supports farmers markets in food desert neighborhoods. These markets offer a wide range of sustainable food options, including locally grown produce, organic products, and culturally diverse offerings. The initiative provides resources to help farmers markets thrive and ensures that they are accessible to all residents, regardless of their socio-economic status.

Furthermore, the Philadelphia Food Justice Initiative focuses on policy advocacy and collaboration with community organizations to address systemic issues that contribute to food deserts. By engaging local stakeholders, including non-profit organizations, government agencies, and residents, the initiative seeks to create a more equitable and sustainable food system.

Conclusion

In the context of food deserts, sustainable food systems and environmental justice are critical considerations. By promoting sustainable practices, such as agroecology and reducing food waste, we can minimize the environmental impact of food production and distribution. Addressing environmental justice ensures that all communities have equitable access to healthy and sustainable food options.

Through community-based approaches, technological solutions, and policy changes, we can work towards creating sustainable food systems in food deserts. By integrating ecological practices and considering environmental justice principles, we can contribute to the overall well-being of communities affected by food deserts, fostering healthier individuals and a more sustainable planet.

Aging and Food Deserts

Nutrition challenges for older adults in food deserts

As we discussed earlier, food deserts are areas where access to healthy and affordable food options is limited. Unfortunately, older adults are particularly vulnerable to the negative impacts of living in food deserts. In this section, we will explore the specific nutrition challenges faced by older adults in food deserts and discuss potential solutions.

Nutritional needs of older adults

Before delving into the challenges, it is important to understand the unique nutritional needs of older adults. As we age, our bodies undergo various physiological changes that affect our nutrient requirements. Older adults often require fewer calories due to decreased metabolism and activity levels. However, their need for essential nutrients such as vitamins, minerals, and protein remains the same or may even increase.

Moreover, older adults are more prone to certain chronic conditions such as heart disease, diabetes, and osteoporosis. These conditions require specific dietary considerations. For example, older adults may need to limit their sodium and sugar intake to manage hypertension and diabetes, respectively.

Limited availability of nutritious food

One of the major nutrition challenges faced by older adults in food deserts is the limited availability of nutritious food. Many food deserts are characterized by an abundance of fast food restaurants and convenience stores, which typically offer processed and unhealthy food options. Fresh fruits, vegetables, and whole grains, which are essential for a balanced diet, are often scarce or not available at all.

Without access to nutritious food, older adults may struggle to meet their recommended daily intake of essential nutrients. This can lead to nutritional deficiencies and increased risk of chronic diseases. For example, inadequate intake of calcium and vitamin D can contribute to the development of osteoporosis in older adults.

Limited mobility and transportation barriers

Another significant challenge faced by older adults in food deserts is limited mobility and transportation barriers. Many older adults rely on public transportation or assistance from others to access grocery stores or supermarkets. However, in food deserts, these options are often limited or non-existent. The lack of reliable and affordable transportation makes it difficult for older adults to travel to places where healthy food options are available.

Additionally, the physical limitations associated with aging, such as decreased mobility and strength, can further exacerbate the problem. Carrying heavy grocery bags or navigating through crowded spaces may be challenging for older adults, making it even more difficult to access nutritious food.

Limited financial resources

Financial constraints also contribute to the nutrition challenges faced by older adults in food deserts. Many older adults live on fixed incomes or rely on social security benefits, which may not be sufficient to afford nutritious food options. Healthy food choices like fresh fruits, vegetables, and lean proteins tend to be more expensive compared to processed and unhealthy alternatives.

As a result, older adults may resort to purchasing cheaper, calorie-dense foods that lack essential nutrients. These food choices can lead to a higher risk of obesity, malnutrition, and chronic diseases.

Solutions and interventions

Addressing the nutrition challenges faced by older adults in food deserts requires a multifaceted approach. Here are some potential solutions and interventions:

- **Improving food access:** Efforts should be made to increase the availability of nutritious food in food deserts. This can include initiatives such as establishing community gardens, farmers markets, and mobile food markets to bring fresh produce directly to the neighborhoods.

- **Transportation assistance:** Providing transportation services specifically targeted towards older adults can help overcome the transportation barriers they face. This can be achieved through collaborations with local transportation authorities or community organizations.

- **Financial support:** Implementing programs that offer financial support or subsidies for older adults to purchase healthy food can help alleviate the financial burden. This can include voucher programs or discounts at local grocery stores or farmers markets.

- **Nutrition education:** Providing nutrition education tailored to the needs of older adults can empower them to make healthier food choices. This can be done through workshops, cooking classes, or nutrition counseling.

- **Community engagement:** Engaging the community and involving older adults in decision-making processes can foster a sense of ownership and empowerment. This can be achieved through community-led initiatives, involvement in designing and implementing interventions, and fostering social connections within the community.

By implementing these solutions, we can strive to improve the nutrition status and overall well-being of older adults living in food deserts. However, it is important to recognize that addressing the nutrition challenges requires a holistic and collaborative effort from policymakers, community organizations, healthcare providers, and individuals themselves.

Let's now explore some real-world examples and case studies of successful interventions in the next subsection.

Case studies of successful interventions

Case Study 1: The Senior Farmers Market Nutrition Program (SFMNP)

The SFMNP is a federally-funded program in the United States that provides eligible older adults with eligible older adults with coupons to purchase fresh fruits, vegetables, herbs, and honey from approved farmers markets, roadside stands, and community-supported agriculture programs. The program aims to increase the consumption of fresh, locally grown produce among older adults while supporting local farmers.

Evaluation of the SFMNP has shown positive outcomes, including increased fruit and vegetable consumption and improved nutritional knowledge among program participants. The program not only addresses the financial barrier but also promotes community engagement and supports local agriculture.

Case Study 2: Community-led food cooperative

In a food desert neighborhood, a group of older adults came together to initiate a community-led food cooperative. The cooperative works by pooling resources, purchasing food in bulk from nearby wholesalers at lower prices, and collectively managing the store. The cooperative provides affordable access to fresh produce, whole grains, and other healthy food options that were previously unavailable in the neighborhood.

This initiative not only ensures nutritious food access but also promotes community engagement, encourages social connections, and empowers older adults to take control of their own food environment.

These are just a few examples of successful interventions that have addressed the nutrition challenges faced by older adults in food deserts. By learning from these examples, we can develop effective strategies to improve the lives of older adults living in these communities.

Summary

In this section, we have explored the specific nutrition challenges faced by older adults in food deserts. Limited availability of nutritious food, limited mobility, transportation barriers, and financial constraints all contribute to the difficulties experienced by older adults in accessing healthy food options. However, various solutions and interventions, such as improving food access, providing transportation assistance, offering financial support, and providing nutrition education, can help address these challenges. By implementing these strategies and learning from successful interventions, we can work towards ensuring that older adults in food deserts have access to the nutritious food they need to maintain their health and well-being.

Health implications of inadequate food access

Access to adequate and nutritious food is essential for maintaining good health. However, in food deserts where there is limited availability of fresh and healthy food options, individuals may face a range of health implications. In this section, we will explore the various health consequences of inadequate food access and the impact it can have on individuals and communities.

Nutritional deficiencies

One of the primary health implications of inadequate food access is the risk of nutritional deficiencies. Food deserts often lack grocery stores and supermarkets that offer a wide variety of fresh fruits, vegetables, whole grains, and lean proteins. As a result, individuals living in these areas may rely on processed and packaged foods that are high in calories, sugar, unhealthy fats, and sodium. These foods contribute to a poor diet lacking essential nutrients such as vitamins, minerals, and fiber.

For example, individuals who do not have access to fresh produce might be deficient in vitamin C and other antioxidants, which are crucial for immune function and overall health. Inadequate intake of vitamins and minerals can lead to compromised immune systems, increased susceptibility to infections, and delayed wound healing.

Obesity and chronic diseases

The lack of access to healthy food options in food deserts is associated with a higher risk of obesity and the development of chronic diseases such as diabetes, cardiovascular diseases, and certain types of cancer. Limited availability of fresh and nutritious food can lead to an overconsumption of energy-dense, nutrient-poor foods, which are often cheaper and more readily available.

A diet high in processed foods, added sugars, and unhealthy fats contributes to weight gain and obesity. Additionally, these types of foods are linked to an increased risk of developing chronic conditions like type 2 diabetes, high blood pressure, and heart diseases. The combination of poor diet and limited physical activity in food deserts further exacerbates these health issues.

Mental health disorders

Food insecurity, which is prevalent in food deserts, has significant psychological impacts on individuals. Living in an environment where reliable access to nutritious food is limited can lead to chronic stress, anxiety, and depression. The uncertainty of food availability and the constant worry about having enough to eat can take a toll on mental well-being.

Furthermore, the lack of variety in food choices can contribute to monotony and dissatisfaction with meals, which can have negative effects on mood and overall mental health. The absence of nutritious foods can also affect cognitive function, memory, and concentration.

Childhood development

Children growing up in food deserts are particularly vulnerable to the health implications of inadequate food access. Proper nutrition during early childhood is critical for optimal growth, brain development, and academic performance. However, limited access to fresh fruits, vegetables, and whole grains can result in inadequate nutrient intake and hinder a child's physical and cognitive development.

Children experiencing food insecurity are more likely to suffer from growth stunting, micronutrient deficiencies, and problems with learning and concentration. These effects can have long-term consequences, impacting academic achievement, earning potential, and overall well-being in adulthood.

Environmental health

The health implications of inadequate food access extend beyond individual well-being to environmental health. Food deserts often lack grocery stores and supermarkets, forcing residents to rely on convenience stores and fast food outlets for their meals. The high consumption of processed foods and fast food contributes to the generation of food packaging waste and pollution.

Additionally, the transportation of food to and within food deserts can contribute to air pollution and greenhouse gas emissions, further impacting environmental health. Addressing food deserts not only improves access to healthy food but also helps in building sustainable and environmentally friendly food systems.

Addressing the health implications

Addressing the health implications of inadequate food access requires a multi-faceted approach involving various stakeholders, including policymakers, community organizations, and individuals themselves. Some potential interventions include:

- Implementing policies to incentivize grocery stores and supermarkets to open in food desert areas, thereby improving access to fresh and nutritious food options.
- Supporting community-based efforts such as urban farming, community gardens, and farmers markets to increase the availability of locally grown produce.
- Utilizing technology, such as mobile apps and online platforms, to connect individuals in food deserts with healthy food options and delivery services.
- Introducing nutrition education programs in schools and communities to promote healthy eating habits and empower individuals with nutrition knowledge.
- Strengthening government assistance programs, such as the Supplemental Nutrition Assistance Program (SNAP), to ensure vulnerable populations have access to affordable and nutritious food.

It is crucial to approach interventions with an equity lens and address the underlying social determinants of food access, such as poverty, inequality, and systemic barriers. By implementing comprehensive solutions and advocating for social justice, we can create lasting change and improve the health outcomes of individuals living in food deserts.

Conclusion

Inadequate food access in food deserts has profound health implications for individuals and communities. Nutritional deficiencies, obesity, chronic diseases, mental health disorders, childhood development issues, and negative environmental impacts are among the various consequences arising from limited access to healthy food options.

To mitigate these health implications, it is essential to adopt a comprehensive approach that addresses the underlying social, economic, and structural factors contributing to food deserts. By implementing policies that promote equitable access to nutritious food, supporting community-based initiatives, utilizing technology, and prioritizing education and health promotion, we can make significant strides towards alleviating the health disparities associated with inadequate food access.

It is incumbent upon all of us, as individuals, communities, and societies, to recognize the importance of food justice and work collectively to ensure that nutritious and affordable food is accessible to all, regardless of their geographical location or socioeconomic status. Only through concerted efforts can we build a healthier and more equitable future for everyone.

Support systems for elderly populations in food deserts

In food deserts, where access to fresh and healthy food is limited, elderly populations face unique challenges in maintaining a nutritious diet. As individuals age, their nutritional needs change, and it becomes even more crucial to ensure they have access to the right types of food. In this section, we will explore the support systems that have been developed to address the specific needs of elderly populations in food deserts.

Elderly individuals often face mobility issues that can make it difficult for them to travel long distances to access grocery stores. Additionally, limited transportation options may further exacerbate the already existing challenges of food deserts. To address these issues, various support systems have been implemented to improve food access for the elderly in food deserts.

One approach is the establishment of mobile food markets targeted specifically at the elderly population. These mobile markets bring fresh produce, pantry staples, and other essential food items directly to the neighborhoods or senior centers where elderly individuals reside. By eliminating the need for transportation, mobile food markets make it easier for seniors to access nutritious options without having to travel long distances.

Another support system for elderly populations in food deserts is the implementation of home delivery services. These services can be coordinated with local grocery stores or community organizations to ensure that elderly individuals receive regular deliveries of fresh and healthy food. This helps seniors overcome transportation barriers and ensures they have a steady supply of nutritious options at their doorstep.

To further support elderly individuals in food deserts, community organizations and non-profit groups have established initiatives to provide assistance with meal preparation. These initiatives often involve volunteers who help seniors with grocery shopping, meal planning, and cooking. By providing practical assistance, these programs not only ensure access to nutritious food but also promote social interaction and companionship, which is important for the overall well-being of the elderly population.

In addition to addressing the immediate need for food access, support systems for elderly populations in food deserts also focus on education and empowerment. Nutrition education programs specifically designed for seniors can help them make informed choices about their diet and understand the importance of balanced nutrition. These programs may include cooking classes, workshops on meal planning, and resources that provide information on healthy eating habits tailored to the needs of older adults.

It is important to recognize that support systems for elderly populations in food deserts should be culturally sensitive and inclusive. A one-size-fits-all approach may not adequately address the diverse needs and preferences of different communities. By involving the elderly population in the decision-making process and tailoring interventions to their specific cultural and dietary preferences, support systems can be more effective and sustainable.

While various support systems have been implemented to address the challenges faced by elderly populations in food deserts, there are still areas for improvement. One challenge is the availability of funding and resources to sustain these initiatives in the long term. Community partnerships, government assistance, and philanthropic efforts can play a crucial role in maintaining and expanding support systems for the elderly.

To evaluate the impact of support systems for elderly populations in food deserts, it is important to consider not only their impact on food access but also their effects on health outcomes and overall well-being. Monitoring indicators such as improved nutrition status, reduced nutritional deficiencies, and increased social engagement can provide insights into the effectiveness of these support systems.

In conclusion, support systems targeting elderly populations in food deserts play a vital role in ensuring that they have access to nutritious food. By addressing barriers to transportation, providing home delivery services, offering meal assistance programs, and promoting nutrition education, these systems help improve the overall well-being of elderly individuals. To ensure their success and sustainability, it is essential to consider the cultural and dietary preferences of the diverse communities and foster collaboration between community organizations, government agencies, and non-profit groups.

Solutions and Interventions for Food Deserts

Policy Changes and Government Initiatives

Legislation addressing food deserts

The issue of food deserts has gained increased attention in recent years, prompting governments to introduce legislation to address this problem. This section will explore some of the key legislation enacted to combat food deserts and improve access to healthy food options.

Healthy Food Financing Initiatives

One approach taken by many governments is the implementation of Healthy Food Financing Initiatives (HFFIs). These initiatives aim to provide financial support and incentives to expand the availability of nutritious foods in underserved communities. The HFFIs typically function through partnerships between government agencies, private businesses, and nonprofit organizations.

One notable example is the Pennsylvania Fresh Food Financing Initiative (FFFI), launched in 2010. The initiative provides grants and loans to food retailers looking to open or renovate supermarkets in underserved areas. Through this program, over 80 fresh food stores have been established or improved, bringing healthier food options to communities that previously lacked access.

Similarly, in the United Kingdom, the Healthy Food Retailer Scheme (HFRS) was introduced. The HFRS provides funding and technical support to retailers, encouraging them to stock and promote healthier food choices. This initiative has helped increase the availability of fresh produce and other nutritious foods in food deserts across the country.

Food Policy Councils

Another legislative approach involves the establishment of Food Policy Councils (FPCs). FPCs are multidisciplinary groups composed of various stakeholders, including government representatives, community organizations, and residents. These councils work together to develop and implement local policies that promote food security and reduce food disparities.

Seattle's Food Action Plan is a pioneering example of how FPCs can address food deserts. The plan aims to improve access to healthy food, increase opportunities for local food production, and promote sustainable agricultural practices. Through partnerships and collaborations, Seattle has successfully implemented programs like Fresh Bucks, which doubles the value of food assistance benefits when used to purchase fresh produce at participating farmers markets.

Zoning and Land-use Regulations

Zoning and land-use regulations can also play a crucial role in addressing food deserts. These regulations can help incentivize the development and maintenance of grocery stores and fresh food retailers in underserved areas.

For instance, in Philadelphia, the city government implemented the Pennsylvania Fresh Food Financing Initiative, as mentioned earlier, in conjunction with zoning changes. These changes allowed for the conversion of vacant lots into supermarkets or grocery stores through streamlined permitting processes and reduced fees. This combination of financial incentives and zoning regulations has played a significant role in increasing access to healthy foods in underserved neighborhoods.

Farmers Market and Mobile Market Support

To promote access to fresh, locally sourced food options, several governments have introduced legislation to support farmers markets and mobile markets.

In the United States, the Farmers Market Promotion Program (FMPP) provides grants to farmers markets and other direct-to-consumer outlets. This funding helps improve infrastructure, enhance marketing efforts, and increase accessibility for underserved populations. By supporting farmers markets in food deserts, the FMPP has contributed to the growth of local, sustainable food systems.

Mobile markets, such as food trucks or buses that bring fresh produce directly to underserved areas, have also gained popularity. In some cases, legislation has been introduced to facilitate and support these initiatives. For example, the Mobile Produce Act in New York City provides funding and resources to mobile market operators, allowing them to offer affordable, high-quality fruits and vegetables to communities lacking access to traditional grocery stores.

Evaluation and Long-term Impact

While legislation addressing food deserts is important, it is equally crucial to evaluate the effectiveness of these interventions over time. Governments should invest in monitoring and research to assess the impact of legislation and make necessary adjustments.

Long-term impact can be evaluated through various measures, including changes in food retail landscapes, improvements in health outcomes, and economic indicators. For example, monitoring the number of supermarkets or grocery stores established in previously underserved areas can provide insights into the success of financing initiatives. Additionally, tracking improvements in health indicators, such as reduced rates of obesity or chronic diseases, can demonstrate the effectiveness of these interventions.

It is important to note that legislation alone may not be sufficient to completely eliminate food deserts. Addressing the underlying social, economic, and environmental factors contributing to food disparities requires a multi-faceted approach that involves various stakeholders and continuous efforts.

Conclusion

Legislation addressing food deserts plays a crucial role in promoting food justice and improving access to healthy, affordable food options. Healthy Food Financing Initiatives, Food Policy Councils, zoning and land-use regulations, and support for farmers markets and mobile markets are just some of the legislative approaches that can help tackle the challenges of food deserts.

Evaluation of the impact of legislation, coupled with a continuous commitment to addressing the complex factors contributing to food deserts, can pave the way for a more equitable food system. Governments, communities, and individuals must work together, leveraging legislation, to build healthier and more sustainable communities and ensure that everyone has access to nutritious foods.

Government-funded programs and initiatives

Government-funded programs and initiatives play a crucial role in addressing food deserts and improving access to nutritious food in underserved communities. These initiatives aim to alleviate food insecurities, promote health equity, and ensure that all individuals have access to affordable and healthy food options. In this section, we will explore some of the major government-funded programs and initiatives that have been implemented to combat food deserts.

Supplemental Nutrition Assistance Program (SNAP)

One significant government-funded program aimed at reducing food insecurity in the United States is the Supplemental Nutrition Assistance Program (SNAP), formerly known as the Food Stamp Program. SNAP provides eligible low-income individuals and families with electronic benefit transfer (EBT) cards, which can be used to purchase food items from authorized retailers, including grocery stores, supermarkets, and farmers markets. The program helps supplement the monthly food budget for millions of Americans, enabling them to purchase a variety of nutritious food items.

SNAP provides recipients with greater food purchasing power, allowing them to make healthier food choices that may have been financially out of reach. The program helps to address the affordability barrier faced by individuals living in food deserts, where healthy food options are often more expensive or less accessible. By providing financial support to eligible individuals, SNAP plays a vital role in bridging the gap between food deserts and nutritious food access.

However, it is important to note that while SNAP is instrumental in addressing food insecurity, it is not specifically designed to target food deserts. Therefore, its impact on improving access to healthy food in underserved areas may vary.

Healthy Food Financing Initiatives

To address the lack of grocery stores and supermarkets in food deserts, various states and local governments have implemented healthy food financing initiatives. These initiatives aim to attract grocery retailers to underserved areas by providing financial incentives such as grants, loans, and tax credits.

For example, Pennsylvania's Fresh Food Financing Initiative (FFFI) provides grants and loans to food retailers to encourage the development of fresh food outlets in low-income communities. The FFFI has successfully incentivized the opening of numerous supermarkets and grocery stores in previously underserved areas, significantly improving access to nutritious food for thousands of individuals.

Similar initiatives have been implemented in other states, such as New York's Healthy Food & Healthy Communities (HFHC) Fund and California's Healthy Food Access Fund. These programs provide financial assistance and technical support to grocery stores and other food retailers looking to establish or expand operations in food deserts. By addressing the financial barriers faced by retailers and incentivizing their presence in underserved areas, these initiatives contribute to reducing food deserts' prevalence and improving food access.

Farmers Market Promotion Program (FMPP)

To support the development and expansion of farmers markets in food deserts, the United States Department of Agriculture (USDA) administers the Farmers Market Promotion Program (FMPP). FMPP provides competitive grants to farmers markets, farm stands, and other direct-to-consumer initiatives to increase access to fresh, healthy, and locally produced food.

The grants awarded through FMPP help farmers markets improve infrastructure, implement marketing strategies, and enhance their ability to accept SNAP benefits. By accepting SNAP and offering a diverse range of locally grown produce, farmers markets become more accessible and appealing to individuals residing in food deserts.

Moreover, FMPP grants facilitate educational activities, such as cooking demonstrations, nutrition workshops, and gardening programs, which aim to promote healthy food choices and increase nutrition knowledge among community members. This multifaceted approach not only enhances food access but also fosters community engagement and empowers individuals to make informed decisions about their food choices.

Healthy Corner Store Initiatives

Another government-funded approach to tackling food deserts involves collaborating with corner stores and small retailers in underserved areas to improve the availability of healthy food options. Healthy Corner Store Initiatives provide financial assistance, technical support, and resources to corner stores to help them offer a wider selection of fresh produce, whole grains, and low-fat dairy products.

For instance, the Healthy Corner Stores Network, funded in part by the Pennsylvania Department of Health, works with corner stores in urban areas to increase access to healthy foods. The program provides assistance in sourcing and displaying fresh produce, creating attractive store layouts, and implementing promotional strategies. These efforts help corner stores overcome logistical and financial barriers associated with stocking and selling fresh food items.

By transforming corner stores into healthier food retailers, these initiatives bring nutritious options closer to individuals living in food deserts. This approach recognizes the existing infrastructure of corner stores and leverages their potential to make a significant impact on improving food access without requiring the establishment of new full-scale grocery stores.

Evaluation and Improvement of Government Programs

As with any government-funded programs, it is crucial to evaluate their effectiveness, identify areas for improvement, and continuously refine the strategies implemented to address food deserts. Evaluations of government programs and initiatives should take into account various factors, including the program's reach, impact, cost-effectiveness, and equity.

One essential aspect of evaluation involves assessing the geographical coverage and accessibility of the programs. It is essential to identify areas that remain underserved despite these initiatives and develop strategies to target them more effectively. This may require adjusting eligibility criteria, expanding outreach efforts, or partnering with community organizations to ensure comprehensive coverage.

Evaluations should also consider the impact of these initiatives on individuals' health outcomes, dietary patterns, and overall well-being. By exploring the association between program participation and health indicators, policymakers can gain valuable insights into the effectiveness of these interventions and identify areas where additional support may be needed.

Furthermore, it is crucial to engage the communities impacted by food deserts in the evaluation process. By soliciting feedback, conducting surveys, and hosting community forums, policymakers can gain firsthand perspectives on the strengths and weaknesses of these initiatives. This inclusive approach helps ensure that the programs meet the specific needs and preferences of the communities they serve.

To continuously improve government programs, it is necessary to incorporate flexibility and adaptability. Staying informed about emerging research, innovative approaches, and best practices in addressing food deserts allows policymakers to update their strategies and optimize their effectiveness.

In summary, government-funded programs and initiatives are pivotal in addressing food deserts and alleviating food insecurity. From SNAP to healthy food financing initiatives, these efforts contribute to improving access to nutritious food, promoting health equity, and empowering individuals to make healthier food choices. By evaluating the impact of these programs and refining their strategies, policymakers can strengthen their effectiveness and strive for a future where food deserts are eliminated entirely.

Evaluation of Policy Effectiveness

Evaluating the effectiveness of policies implemented to address food deserts is crucial in understanding their impact and making informed decisions about future interventions. This section explores the methods and metrics used to measure the success of such policies, highlighting the importance of monitoring food access and availability, assessing health outcomes and behavior changes, and considering social and economic indicators of progress.

Monitoring Food Access and Availability

One key aspect of evaluating policy effectiveness is monitoring food access and availability in areas targeted by interventions. This involves assessing the presence and proximity of grocery stores, supermarkets, farmers markets, and other sources of fresh and healthy food within food desert communities. A common approach is to use Geographic Information System (GIS) mapping to visually represent the distribution and density of food retail outlets.

To complement GIS mapping, researchers and policymakers often conduct on-the-ground surveys and interviews to gather qualitative data on residents' experiences and perceptions of food access. These surveys may include questions about travel distance to the nearest grocery store, perceived affordability and variety of healthy food options, and barriers faced when trying to access nutritious food. Such qualitative data provide valuable insights into the lived experiences of individuals affected by food deserts and can inform policy decisions.

Assessing Health Outcomes and Behavior Changes

Evaluating policy effectiveness also requires assessing changes in health outcomes and behaviors following the implementation of interventions. Some key health indicators include changes in rates of obesity, diabetes, and cardiovascular diseases, as well as improvements in overall diet quality and nutrient intake.

Researchers often rely on data from national health surveys and electronic health records to track changes in these health outcomes over time. Additionally, randomized controlled trials (RCTs) and quasi-experimental studies may be conducted to measure the impact of specific interventions on health behaviors and outcomes. For example, an RCT could compare the health outcomes of individuals living in food deserts who receive subsidies for purchasing healthy foods with those who do not receive any support.

In addition to assessing individual-level health outcomes, it is important to consider the broader community-level impacts of interventions. For instance, policies aimed at increasing access to healthy food may have spillover effects on community engagement, social cohesion, and collective efforts to address food insecurity.

Considering Social and Economic Indicators of Progress

While improvements in food access and health outcomes are critical measures of policy effectiveness, it is also essential to consider social and economic indicators to evaluate the broader impact of interventions. Key indicators to consider include changes in employment rates, income levels, poverty rates, and educational attainment within food desert communities.

Evaluating the economic impact of policies helps assess the effectiveness of measures taken to address the underlying socioeconomic factors contributing to food deserts. For example, policies that create job opportunities in food retail or support local food production can have positive effects on employment and income levels. Similarly, initiatives that promote nutrition education and improve access to educational resources can contribute to increased educational attainment and empowerment within these communities.

Social indicators such as community engagement, social capital, and social cohesion should also be considered. Policies that foster community participation, collaboration, and empowerment in addressing food deserts can have long-lasting and sustainable impacts.

Conclusion

Evaluating the effectiveness of policies aimed at addressing food deserts is essential for understanding their impact and making informed decisions about future interventions. By monitoring food access and availability, assessing health outcomes and behavior changes, and considering social and economic indicators of progress, policymakers can gain valuable insights into the effectiveness of their interventions. This knowledge can inform the design and implementation of evidence-based policies that effectively tackle the issue of food deserts and promote equitable access to healthy food for all.

Community-Based Approaches

Community gardens and urban farming

Community gardens and urban farming are emerging as effective solutions for addressing food deserts. These initiatives involve the cultivation of fruits, vegetables, and herbs in shared spaces within urban areas, with the primary goal of increasing access to fresh and nutritious produce. In this section, we will explore the principles and benefits of community gardens and urban farming, as well as provide examples of successful projects and strategies for implementing these interventions.

Principles of Community Gardens

Community gardens are cooperative ventures where individuals, families, or organizations collectively cultivate and maintain plots of land. These gardens are typically located in urban areas where green spaces are limited, making them highly accessible for community members. The principles that guide community gardens include:

1. **Shared ownership and management:** Community gardens are owned and managed collectively by the participants, fostering a sense of ownership, responsibility, and community cohesion.
2. **Sustainable practices:** Gardens often prioritize organic farming techniques, such as composting, water conservation, and minimizing the use of chemical fertilizers and pesticides. This approach promotes environmental sustainability and healthier growing methods.
3. **Education and skill-sharing:** Community gardens provide a platform for sharing knowledge and expertise in gardening, nutrition, and sustainable practices. Participants can learn from one another and develop valuable skills that can be applied beyond the garden.
4. **Social engagement:** Gardens serve as meeting places for community members, promoting social interaction, and fostering relationships. They become hubs for community events, workshops, and social activities that promote social cohesion and a sense of belonging.

Benefits of Community Gardens

Community gardens and urban farming have numerous benefits for individuals, communities, and the environment. Some key benefits include:

1. **Improved access to fresh produce:** By cultivating their own fruits and vegetables, community gardeners have a consistent supply of fresh and nutritious food. This reduces their reliance on convenience stores and increases their access to a variety of seasonal produce.

2. **Healthier food choices:** Community gardens encourage participants to incorporate more fruits and vegetables into their diets, leading to improved nutrition and better overall health. Access to fresh produce promotes healthier eating habits, reducing the risk of diet-related diseases.

3. **Enhanced mental well-being:** Gardening has been shown to have positive effects on mental health, reducing stress and anxiety. It provides a therapeutic and calming environment, allowing individuals to connect with nature and reap the psychological benefits of spending time outdoors.

4. **Environmental sustainability:** Community gardens promote sustainable agricultural practices, such as composting and water conservation. They also contribute to urban greening, improving air quality and mitigating the effects of climate change.

5. **Educational opportunities:** Community gardens serve as living classrooms, providing education on sustainable agriculture, nutrition, and environmental stewardship. This empowers community members to make informed choices about their food and the environment.

Successful Examples and Strategies

Numerous community garden initiatives have demonstrated success in addressing food deserts and promoting community well-being. Here are a few examples and strategies that have yielded positive results:

1. **The Green Thumb Initiative (GTI):** This project, based in a low-income neighborhood, transformed abandoned lots into thriving community gardens. GTI engaged community members in all aspects of garden management, providing training on organic farming, nutrition education, and entrepreneurship. This initiative not only increased food access but also created job opportunities and improved community resilience.

2. **Urban Agriculture Cooperative:** By establishing an urban farming cooperative, community members can collectively manage larger-scale agricultural projects. This cooperative model allows for increased productivity and resource sharing, resulting in a more sustainable and economically viable urban farming system.

3. **Youth Engagement Programs:** Community gardens that involve young people not only teach them valuable skills but also instill a sense of ownership and

responsibility. These programs offer mentorship and educational opportunities, empowering youth to become leaders in their communities and advocates for sustainable food systems.

Implementing Community Gardens

Implementing community gardens requires careful planning, collaboration, and support. Some key considerations for establishing successful community gardens include:

1. **Identify suitable locations:** Look for available land, such as unused lots, parks, or school grounds, ideally in or near food deserts. Secure permission from landowners and evaluate the soil quality and sunlight availability for gardening.
2. **Community engagement:** Engage community members from the outset to ensure their involvement and ownership. Conduct community meetings, workshops, and surveys to assess interest, gather input, and build support for the project.
3. **Collaborate with local organizations:** Partner with local nonprofits, schools, government agencies, and businesses for funding, technical assistance, and expertise. Collaboration strengthens community ties and broadens available resources.
4. **Provide necessary resources:** Ensure access to water, gardening tools, seeds, compost, and other essential resources. Seek grants, donations, and sponsorships from local businesses or organizations to support these needs.
5. **Establish a management plan:** Develop a clear organizational structure for the community garden, including rules for plot allocation, maintenance responsibilities, and decision-making processes. Encourage regular communication, collaboration, and accountability among participants.
6. **Promote education and outreach:** Offer workshops, training sessions, and educational programs on gardening techniques, nutrition, and sustainability. Engage local schools and community organizations to integrate the garden into their curricula and activities.
7. **Ensure long-term sustainability:** Develop strategies for ongoing maintenance, funding, and community involvement. Consider options such as volunteer programs, farmers markets, or selling surplus produce to sustain the garden's operations.

Conclusion

Community gardens and urban farming offer practical and empowering solutions for combating food deserts. They provide communities with access to fresh and nutritious food, promote sustainable practices, strengthen community bonds, and offer educational opportunities. By implementing strategies for community engagement, resource mobilization, and capacity building, community gardens can create lasting impacts and pave the way for a more equitable and sustainable food system.

In the next section, we will explore the role of farmers markets and food cooperatives in addressing food deserts.

Farmers Markets and Food Cooperatives

Farmers markets and food cooperatives are two community-based approaches that can help address the issue of food deserts. These initiatives aim to improve food access by providing fresh, healthy, and locally produced food options. In this section, we will explore the concept and benefits of farmers markets and food cooperatives, their role in promoting food justice, and their potential challenges.

Farmers Markets

Farmers markets are physical spaces where local farmers, growers, and producers gather to sell their fresh produce directly to consumers. These markets offer a range of fruits, vegetables, meats, dairy products, baked goods, and other locally sourced items. They provide an opportunity for consumers to connect with farmers and learn about the origin and production methods of the food they buy.

One of the primary advantages of farmers markets in food desert areas is the availability of fresh and seasonal produce. Unlike chain supermarkets, which often stock produce that needs to be transported long distances and may lack nutritional quality, farmers markets offer locally grown fruits and vegetables that are picked at their peak ripeness. This ensures that consumers have access to nutritious food options that are both flavorful and sustainable.

In addition to providing fresh food, farmers markets also contribute to the local economy. By supporting local farmers and small-scale producers, money circulates within the community, creating opportunities for economic growth and job creation. Farmers markets can also serve as platforms for entrepreneurial initiatives, enabling new farmers or food entrepreneurs to start their businesses and introduce innovative products.

Furthermore, farmers markets foster a sense of community and social interaction. They provide a vibrant space for people to gather, exchange ideas, and build relationships. Community members can engage in conversations with farmers, ask questions about farming practices, and receive advice on cooking and meal planning. This direct connection between consumers and producers not only enhances the overall shopping experience but also promotes transparency and trust in the food system.

However, farmers markets may face several challenges in food desert areas. One significant issue is the affordability of fresh produce. In low-income communities, the cost of locally grown and organic food may be higher than the heavily subsidized processed foods available at chain supermarkets. This financial barrier can limit the accessibility of farmers markets to certain populations. To address this challenge, farmers markets can partner with government programs, such as the Supplemental Nutrition Assistance Program (SNAP), to accept EBT cards and offer discounts to low-income individuals.

Another challenge is the limited availability and seasonality of certain produce items. Farmers markets predominantly offer locally sourced products, which means that certain fruits and vegetables may only be available during specific months due to regional growing seasons. Additionally, farmers markets may not have a wide range of culturally specific foods that cater to diverse communities. Efforts should be made to diversify the produce offerings and extend the availability of fresh food throughout the year through collaborations with local farmers and regional agricultural initiatives.

To overcome these challenges and ensure the success of farmers markets in food desert areas, collaboration and support from various stakeholders are essential. Local governments can provide financial incentives and technical assistance to farmers markets, such as offering affordable spaces, organizing outreach campaigns, and facilitating partnerships. Non-profit organizations, community groups, and volunteers can also play a crucial role in promoting farmers markets and advocating for their establishment in underserved neighborhoods.

Food Cooperatives

Food cooperatives, also known as co-ops, are member-owned grocery stores that operate based on the principles of shared ownership, democratic decision-making, and community involvement. These cooperative models aim to provide affordable and healthy food options to their members, while also prioritizing social and environmental sustainability.

Unlike traditional grocery stores, food cooperatives emphasize transparency, ethical sourcing, and supporting local farmers and producers. Members typically pay an annual fee and have a say in the store's governance, including decisions related to product selection, pricing, and community programs. By collectively pooling resources and sharing the risks and benefits, cooperatives can offer high-quality food at lower prices compared to for-profit supermarkets.

Food cooperatives are particularly well-suited for addressing the needs of food deserts because they prioritize community engagement and cooperation. They often emerge in response to the lack of accessible and affordable grocery stores in underserved areas. By involving community members directly in the operation of the store, food cooperatives foster a sense of ownership and agency, empowering individuals to take control of their food environment.

In addition to providing affordable and healthy food options, food cooperatives often prioritize sourcing products from local farmers and producers. This not only supports the local economy but also reduces the carbon footprint associated with long-distance transportation. Many food cooperatives have commitments to organic farming practices, fair trade, and environmentally sustainable packaging, further promoting sustainable and ethical food systems.

While food cooperatives can be effective in addressing food deserts, they also face challenges. One common barrier is the initial financial investment required to establish a cooperative store. Securing funding, finding suitable premises, and navigating legal and administrative procedures can be complex and time-consuming. However, cooperatives can seek support through grants, loans, and partnerships with local organizations or municipalities that are invested in addressing food inequities.

Cooperative education and member engagement are another critical aspect of successful food cooperatives. To ensure ongoing participation and commitment, cooperatives need to provide opportunities for member education, training, and involvement in decision-making processes. This can be achieved through workshops, cooking classes, food demos, and regular general assemblies where members can voice their opinions and contribute to shaping the cooperative's policies and practices.

Food cooperatives can also face challenges related to scale and growth. As the cooperative expands and serves a larger number of members, it needs to maintain a balance between financial sustainability and accessibility. Cooperatives must strike a balance between keeping prices affordable and ensuring the long-term viability of the store. This requires effective financial management, strategic planning, and continuous engagement with members and the broader community.

Overall, farmers markets and food cooperatives are community-driven approaches that have the potential to make a significant impact on food deserts. By providing fresh, locally sourced food options at affordable prices, these initiatives empower individuals, strengthen social connections, and contribute to sustainable and equitable food systems. To ensure their success, collaboration, and support from various stakeholders, including governments, non-profit organizations, and community members, are crucial. By working together, we can create a more just and inclusive food system for all.

Collaborative Efforts and Community Empowerment

Collaborative efforts and community empowerment play a crucial role in addressing food deserts and improving access to healthy food options. By engaging community members, organizations, and stakeholders, these initiatives can lead to sustainable solutions that are tailored to the specific needs of the community. This section will explore the various collaborative approaches and strategies that have been successful in empowering communities and creating positive change.

Community Engagement and Participation

One of the key principles of collaborative efforts is the active involvement of the community in problem-solving and decision-making processes. Community engagement ensures that the voices and perspectives of the people affected by food deserts are taken into account. It fosters a sense of ownership and empowerment among community members, as they become active participants in finding solutions to the challenges they face.

To promote community engagement, it is important to create opportunities for open dialogue and meaningful participation. This can be achieved through town hall meetings, focus groups, or community forums where residents can express their concerns, share their experiences, and contribute their ideas. By listening to community members, policymakers and organizations can gain valuable insights into the specific barriers and needs of the community.

Collaborative Partnerships

Creating collaborative partnerships between various stakeholders is essential for the success of efforts to address food deserts. These partnerships bring together individuals, organizations, businesses, and government entities that have a vested interest in improving food access and promoting community health. By pooling resources, expertise, and networks, collaborative partnerships can leverage collective strengths to drive sustainable solutions.

Examples of collaborative partners include local government agencies, nonprofit organizations, community health centers, farmers, grocery stores, and educational institutions. Each partner brings unique perspectives and resources to the table, allowing for a comprehensive approach to tackling food deserts. For example, a partnership between a nonprofit organization, a local government agency, and a farmers' cooperative could work together to establish a farmers market in a food desert, providing fresh and affordable produce to the community.

Capacity Building and Skill Development

Collaborative efforts and community empowerment should not only focus on short-term interventions but also aim to build long-term capacity within the community. This involves equipping community members with the knowledge, skills, and resources needed to sustain and expand initiatives addressing food deserts.

Capacity building efforts may include workshops and training sessions on topics such as nutrition education, gardening, food entrepreneurship, and advocacy. These activities empower individuals to take control of their own health and well-being, and often lead to the development of new local food businesses or community-led initiatives.

For example, a community garden project in a food desert can not only provide fresh produce but also serve as a platform for educational programs. Residents can learn gardening skills, healthy cooking techniques, and even start their own small-scale farming enterprises. These initiatives not only address immediate food access issues but also foster economic opportunities and self-sufficiency within the community.

Reaching Underserved Populations

Collaborative efforts should be inclusive and ensure that underserved populations within food deserts are not left behind. This includes reaching out to marginalized communities such as low-income households, racial and ethnic minorities, elderly individuals, and individuals with disabilities.

To effectively reach these populations, it is important to consider cultural sensitivities, language barriers, and specific needs. Collaborative efforts can involve partnering with community-based organizations that have established trust and rapport with these communities. For example, engaging community leaders, religious institutions, and local grassroots organizations can help bridge the gap and ensure that initiatives are designed and implemented in a culturally appropriate manner.

Evaluation and Continuous Improvement

Collaborative efforts and community empowerment should be based on evidence-based practices and rigorous evaluation to ensure their effectiveness. This involves monitoring and measuring the impact of interventions, identifying areas for improvement, and making data-driven decisions.

Evaluation can be done through various methods such as surveys, interviews, focus groups, and analysis of health and economic indicators. By collecting feedback from community members and stakeholders, it becomes possible to assess the success of interventions and make necessary adjustments.

Collaborative efforts should also allow for continuous learning and adaptation. This means recognizing that no single solution will fit all communities and being open to experimenting with different approaches. Sharing best practices and lessons learned across communities and organizations can further enhance the impact of collaborative efforts.

Conclusion

Collaborative efforts and community empowerment are essential for addressing food deserts and improving access to healthy food options. By involving community members, creating partnerships, building capacity, and reaching underserved populations, these initiatives can have a lasting impact on the health and well-being of communities.

It is important to recognize that addressing food deserts requires a multifaceted approach. Collaborative efforts should be supported by policy changes, investment in infrastructure, and targeted funding to ensure long-term sustainability. By working together, communities, organizations, and policymakers can create a future where everyone has access to nutritious and affordable food, regardless of their geographic location or socioeconomic status.

Technological Solutions

Mobile apps and online platforms

Mobile apps and online platforms have emerged as valuable tools in addressing the issue of food deserts. These technological advancements have the potential to improve access to nutritious food, enhance food choices, and empower individuals to make informed decisions about their diet. This section explores the various ways in which mobile apps and online platforms can contribute to addressing food deserts, their benefits, challenges, and potential future developments.

Benefits of Mobile apps and online platforms

Mobile apps and online platforms offer several benefits in addressing the challenges faced by food desert communities.

Firstly, these tools can provide valuable information about the availability and accessibility of healthy food options in the area. Users can easily find nearby grocery stores, farmers markets, food pantries, and other sources of fresh and affordable produce. These apps and platforms can also provide detailed information about the products available, including nutritional content, ingredient lists, and pricing, enabling users to make informed choices.

Secondly, mobile apps and online platforms can help bridge the transportation gap in food deserts. By providing access to food delivery services, users can order groceries and have them delivered directly to their doorstep, eliminating the need for reliable transportation to access healthy food options.

Thirdly, these tools can facilitate community engagement and collaboration. Users can connect with each other to share information, resources, and experiences related to finding and utilizing healthy food options. Online platforms can also host forums, discussion groups, and social media spaces where community members can share recipes, cooking tips, and other food-related knowledge.

Challenges and limitations

While mobile apps and online platforms offer promising solutions, they also come with challenges and limitations that need to be addressed.

One key challenge is the digital divide, which refers to the gap in internet access and technological literacy among different populations. In low-income communities and among certain demographic groups, access to smartphones and reliable internet may be limited. Therefore, efforts should be made to ensure equitable access to these tools, such as providing public Wi-Fi and digital literacy training.

Another challenge is the accuracy and reliability of information provided by mobile apps and online platforms. It is crucial to ensure that the information about food sources, prices, and nutritional content is up-to-date and verified. Additionally, attention should be given to the design and usability of these tools, making sure they are user-friendly and accessible to individuals with diverse technological skills and abilities.

Examples of mobile apps and online platforms

Several existing mobile apps and online platforms have made significant strides in addressing food deserts. Here are a few examples:

- **Goodr:** Goodr is a mobile app that connects food businesses with surplus food to local organizations and individuals in need. It reduces food waste by redirecting excess food to communities experiencing food insecurity.

- **UrbanSitter:** UrbanSitter is an online platform that connects parents with local babysitters and nannies. By offering reliable childcare options, it enables parents in food deserts to have more flexibility in accessing healthy food options outside their neighborhoods.

- **FreshEBT:** FreshEBT is a mobile app that allows users to check their Electronic Benefits Transfer (EBT) food stamp balance and find stores that accept EBT. This app helps individuals in low-income communities better manage their food assistance benefits.

These examples demonstrate the diverse ways in which mobile apps and online platforms can support food desert communities, from reducing food waste and increasing access to affordable childcare to improving the utilization of government assistance programs.

Future developments

The future of mobile apps and online platforms in addressing food deserts holds great promise. Here are some potential developments to watch for:

- **Personalized nutrition recommendations:** Advances in data analytics and machine learning may enable the development of mobile apps that provide personalized nutrition recommendations based on individual needs, preferences, and health conditions. This could help individuals make healthier food choices tailored to their specific circumstances.

- **Virtual reality experiences:** Virtual reality (VR) technology can be utilized to provide immersive experiences that simulate grocery shopping or provide culinary training. By bringing the shopping experience or cooking demonstrations directly to users, VR technology can help overcome the physical barriers of food access.

- **Collaborative online platforms:** Building on the success of existing online platforms, future developments may focus on fostering collaboration and co-creation among community members. These platforms could facilitate collective decision-making, resource sharing, and community-led initiatives to address food deserts.

These potential developments highlight the exciting possibilities that lie ahead in utilizing mobile apps and online platforms to tackle the complex issue of food deserts.

Summary

Mobile apps and online platforms offer innovative solutions to address the challenges faced by food deserts. They provide information on food availability, bridge transportation gaps, and foster community engagement. Despite the challenges of the digital divide and ensuring information accuracy, these tools have demonstrated their potential in improving food access. Examples such as Goodr, UrbanSitter, and FreshEBT showcase their diverse applications. Looking ahead, personalized nutrition recommendations, virtual reality experiences, and collaborative online platforms hold promise for future developments in addressing food deserts. By leveraging the power of technology, we can make significant strides in promoting equitable access to healthy food for all communities.

Food delivery services in food deserts

Food delivery services have emerged as a potential solution to address the lack of access to fresh and healthy foods in food deserts. These services aim to provide convenient and reliable delivery of groceries and other food items to individuals living in these underserved areas. In this section, we will explore the concept of food delivery services in food deserts, the challenges they face, and their potential impact on improving food access and nutrition.

The need for food delivery services in food deserts

In food deserts, residents often face numerous barriers to accessing healthy foods, such as limited transportation options, long distances to grocery stores, and a lack of affordable fresh produce. These challenges contribute to a cycle of poor nutrition and negative health outcomes within these communities. Food delivery services have the potential to alleviate some of these barriers by bringing fresh food directly to the doorsteps of individuals who would otherwise struggle to access it.

Operating models of food delivery services

There are different operating models for food delivery services in food deserts, each with its own strengths and limitations. Let's explore three common models:

1. Non-profit organizations: Some non-profit organizations have started food delivery initiatives specifically designed for low-income communities. They rely on grants, donations, and partnerships with local farmers and grocery stores to source the food. These services often prioritize affordability and accessibility, offering subsidized or discounted prices for customers in need.

2. Local grocery store delivery: In this model, existing grocery stores partner with delivery services or develop their own delivery infrastructure to serve customers in food desert areas. Customers can place their grocery orders online or through a mobile app, and the deliveries are scheduled at regular intervals. This model leverages existing infrastructure and supply chains, making it a cost-effective option.

3. Independent delivery services: Independent companies have also emerged, specializing in delivering groceries to food desert communities. These companies often focus on sourcing fresh and local produce and may offer a wider range of food options compared to traditional grocery stores. They typically operate on a subscription or on-demand basis, allowing customers to customize their orders and delivery schedules.

Challenges and considerations

While food delivery services show promise in addressing food access issues in food deserts, several challenges need to be considered:

1. Delivery costs: The cost of delivering groceries to remote or underserved areas can be higher than in more densely populated regions. This cost can be a significant barrier to the sustainability of food delivery services, especially for non-profit organizations operating on tight budgets.

2. Infrastructure limitations: Food deserts often lack the necessary infrastructure to support efficient delivery services, such as reliable roads, transportation networks, and adequate cold storage facilities. Overcoming these infrastructure limitations can be a challenge for food delivery initiatives.

3. Digital divide: Many individuals in food deserts may not have access to smartphones, computers, or reliable internet connections, making it difficult for them to take advantage of online ordering and delivery services. Addressing the digital divide is crucial to ensure equitable access to food delivery services.

Impact of food delivery services

Despite the challenges, food delivery services have the potential to make a significant impact on improving food access and nutrition in food deserts. Some of the potential benefits include:

1. Increased access to fresh and healthy food: By delivering groceries directly to people's homes, food delivery services overcome transportation barriers and provide individuals in food deserts with convenient access to fresh produce, whole grains, and other nutritious food items.

2. Expansion of food choices: Food delivery services can offer a wider variety of food options compared to the limited selection available in traditional brick-and-mortar grocery stores in food deserts. This can empower individuals to make healthier choices and diversify their diets.

3. Opportunities for local sourcing: Many food delivery services prioritize sourcing food from local farmers and suppliers. This not only supports local economies but also promotes sustainable agricultural practices and strengthens the local food system.

Case study: "FreshRoutes"

One example of a food delivery service in a food desert is the "FreshRoutes" program in Philadelphia, USA. FreshRoutes operates as a non-profit mobile produce market, using retrofitted school buses as mobile grocery stores. They visit pre-determined locations within low-income neighborhoods, allowing residents to purchase fresh produce and other groceries directly from the bus. The program partners with local farmers and grocery stores to ensure a diverse range of nutritious food options.

Conclusion

Food delivery services have the potential to address some of the challenges associated with food deserts by delivering fresh and healthy foods directly to individuals' doorsteps. While they face challenges such as high delivery costs and infrastructure limitations, these services can increase access to nutritious food, expand food choices, and support local economies. Moving forward, it is important to consider strategies to overcome these challenges and support the sustainable growth of food delivery services in food deserts.

Using technology to bridge the food access gap

In recent years, technological advancements have provided new opportunities to address the issue of food deserts and bridge the food access gap. Through the use of various technologies, innovative solutions have emerged to improve access to healthy and affordable food in underserved communities. In this section, we will explore some of these technological interventions and their potential to make a significant impact.

Online platforms and mobile apps

One of the key ways technology is being used to address food deserts is through the development of online platforms and mobile applications. These platforms serve as virtual marketplaces that connect consumers in food deserts with local farmers, grocery stores, and food suppliers. By providing an online platform for ordering and delivering groceries, these apps enable residents of food deserts to access a wider range of fresh and healthy food options.

For example, the "Fresh to Door" app allows users to order fresh produce and groceries from local farmers and have them delivered directly to their homes. The app also provides information on nutrition and healthy eating habits, empowering users to make informed food choices. Similarly, the "Food Finder" app connects users with nearby grocery stores and farmers markets, helping them find the closest and most affordable options for fresh produce.

These online platforms and mobile apps not only bridge the physical distance between consumers and food retailers but also help alleviate the transportation challenges often associated with food deserts. By providing convenient and efficient delivery options, these technological solutions enable residents to overcome barriers related to transportation and mobility.

Food delivery services

In addition to online platforms and mobile apps, food delivery services have emerged as a promising solution for improving food access in underserved areas. These services partner with local grocery stores, farmers markets, and restaurants to deliver fresh and healthy food directly to consumers' doorsteps.

One notable example is the "Fresh Express" program, which collaborates with grocery stores and farmers markets to deliver pre-packed boxes of fresh produce and other essential food items to residents of food deserts. These boxes are often provided at subsidized prices, making them more affordable for low-income individuals and families. By bringing the food directly to the consumers, food delivery services eliminate the need for transportation and enable individuals to access nutritious food without leaving their homes.

Furthermore, some food delivery services have incorporated innovative technologies to enhance efficiency and accessibility. For instance, drones are being tested as a means of delivering groceries to remote and inaccessible areas. This technology has the potential to revolutionize food delivery in rural and geographically isolated food deserts, where conventional transportation infrastructure may be lacking.

Smart vending machines and kiosks

Smart vending machines and kiosks have also emerged as a technological innovation to bridge the food access gap. These machines are strategically placed in food deserts, providing convenient and accessible options for purchasing fresh produce, healthy snacks, and ready-to-eat meals.

What sets smart vending machines apart from traditional vending machines is their ability to offer healthier and more nutritious options. These machines are stocked with a variety of fresh fruits, vegetables, whole-grain products, and low-sugar beverages. Moreover, they often provide nutritional information and healthy cooking tips to educate consumers about making healthier choices.

Additionally, smart vending machines can be equipped with cashless payment systems, such as mobile payment apps, to ensure accessibility for individuals who may not have access to traditional banking services. By combining convenience, accessibility, and healthier food options, smart vending machines help address the problem of food deserts in a user-friendly and cost-effective manner.

Community refrigerators

A unique and community-driven solution to address food deserts is the concept of community refrigerators. These are shared refrigerators that are placed in public spaces, allowing individuals and businesses to donate and access surplus food. Community members can contribute fresh produce, leftovers from restaurants, or excess groceries to these refrigerators, making them available to those in need.

Technology can play a role in the management and coordination of community refrigerators. For example, mobile apps can be developed to provide real-time information about the availability of food items in these refrigerators, helping users plan their visits more effectively. These apps can also incorporate features that allow individuals to request specific food items, fostering a sense of community engagement and collaboration.

Community refrigerators not only address the immediate need for food access but also promote sustainability by reducing food waste. They provide a platform for individuals and businesses to contribute to the well-being of their community and ensure that nutritious food is not wasted but rather made accessible to those who need it.

Conclusion

Technology has the potential to play a significant role in bridging the food access gap in food deserts. Online platforms, mobile apps, food delivery services, smart vending machines, and community refrigerators are all examples of innovative technological interventions that can improve food access, promote healthier food choices, and empower underserved communities.

However, it is important to note that technological solutions alone cannot fully address the underlying systemic issues that contribute to food deserts. Access to technology itself may be limited in some communities, particularly among low-income populations. Additionally, addressing the root causes of food deserts, such as poverty, transportation barriers, and lack of economic opportunities, requires a comprehensive and multi-pronged approach.

Therefore, while technology has the potential to be a valuable tool in bridging the food access gap, it should be seen as a complement to broader social, economic, and policy interventions. By combining technological innovation with community engagement, policy changes, and advocacy efforts, we can work towards a future where everyone has equitable access to healthy and affordable food, regardless of their geographic location or socioeconomic status.

Education and Health Promotion

Nutrition education in schools and communities

Nutrition education plays a crucial role in addressing food deserts and improving the overall health and well-being of individuals in schools and communities. By providing knowledge and skills related to healthy eating, nutrition education empowers individuals to make informed food choices and promotes healthy behaviors. This section will explore the importance of nutrition education, discuss effective approaches to delivering nutrition education in schools and communities, and provide examples of successful programs.

Importance of nutrition education

Nutrition education is essential because it equips individuals with the knowledge and skills needed to make healthy food choices. It teaches individuals about the importance of a balanced diet, the role of different nutrients in the body, and the impact of food choices on overall health. By understanding nutrition concepts, individuals can make informed decisions about what they eat, leading to improved dietary habits and better health outcomes.

In a food desert context, where healthy food options are limited, nutrition education becomes even more critical. It empowers individuals to maximize their available resources and make the most nutritious choices possible. By learning how to navigate food labels, plan balanced meals, and prepare healthy recipes with limited ingredients, individuals in food deserts can overcome the challenges they face and improve their nutritional status.

Approaches to delivering nutrition education

There are several effective approaches to delivering nutrition education in schools and communities. These approaches range from classroom-based interventions to community-based programs, each with its unique advantages.

In schools, incorporating nutrition education into the curriculum is a common approach. This can be done through dedicated health or science classes, integrating nutrition concepts into other subjects like math and biology, or implementing school-wide wellness initiatives. By making nutrition education a part of the regular curriculum, schools provide consistent and structured opportunities for students to learn about healthy eating.

Community-based programs also play a significant role in delivering nutrition education. These programs can be conducted by local health departments, non-profit organizations, or community centers. They can take the form of workshops, cooking demonstrations, grocery store tours, or gardening programs. By engaging with the community directly, these programs can address the specific needs and challenges individuals face in food deserts, making the education more relevant and impactful.

Examples of successful programs

There are several successful nutrition education programs that have been implemented in schools and communities to address food deserts. These programs serve as models for effective approaches and provide valuable insights into best practices.

One such program is the "Farm to School" initiative, which brings locally grown, fresh produce into school cafeterias and incorporates nutrition education into the curriculum. By connecting students with healthy food options and teaching them about the source of their food, this program promotes healthy eating habits and encourages a greater appreciation for fresh, local produce.

Another successful program is the "Cooking Matters" campaign, which offers hands-on cooking classes and nutrition education to low-income families. The program aims to improve cooking skills, increase food knowledge, and empower families to make healthy choices on a limited budget. By providing practical skills and resources, Cooking Matters equips families in food deserts to overcome barriers and prioritize nutrition.

The "Healthy Corner Store Initiative" is another example of a successful program that focuses on community-based nutrition education. This initiative transforms small corner stores in food deserts into sources of healthy food options. Through partnerships with local businesses, the program offers nutrition education, recipe demonstrations, and support for store owners to stock fresh produce and healthier snacks. This approach not only improves access to nutritious food but also empowers the community to make healthier choices.

Challenges and considerations

While nutrition education programs have proven to be effective, several challenges and considerations need to be addressed to ensure their success. One challenge is the need for cultural relevance and sensitivity. Food choices and dietary preferences are often deeply rooted in cultural traditions, and any nutrition education program must respect and acknowledge these cultural differences. By incorporating culturally appropriate recipes, ingredients, and cooking techniques, programs can ensure that the education provided is relevant and meaningful to the community.

Another challenge is the need for ongoing support and follow-up. Nutrition education is not a one-time event but rather a continuous process. Individuals need consistent reinforcement and guidance to sustain healthy behaviors. Therefore, programs should consider incorporating periodic check-ins, support groups, or follow-up sessions to provide ongoing support and monitor progress.

Lastly, it is essential to involve key stakeholders, such as parents, teachers, community leaders, and local policymakers, in the planning and implementation of nutrition education programs. By engaging these stakeholders, programs can gain support, resources, and a broader impact. Additionally, involving the community in decision-making processes ensures that the programs are tailored to the specific needs and cultural context of the target population.

Conclusion

Nutrition education in schools and communities is a powerful tool for addressing food deserts and promoting healthy eating habits. By providing individuals with the knowledge and skills necessary to make informed food choices, nutrition education empowers individuals to overcome the challenges of limited food access and improve their overall health outcomes. Through effective approaches, such as integrating nutrition education into the curriculum, implementing community-based programs, and leveraging successful models, we can create a future where everyone has equal access to healthy food options and the knowledge to make nourishing choices.

Public health campaigns in food deserts

In tackling the issue of food deserts, public health campaigns play a crucial role in raising awareness, promoting healthy behaviors, and advocating for change. Public health campaigns aim to educate individuals and communities about the importance of nutrition, provide information on available resources, and empower individuals to make healthier choices. In this section, we will explore the strategies and approaches used in public health campaigns targeting food deserts, as well as the challenges and opportunities they present.

The Role of Public Health in Addressing Food Deserts

Public health plays a vital role in addressing the health disparities associated with food deserts. By focusing on prevention and health promotion, public health campaigns seek to address the underlying social, economic, and environmental factors contributing to food deserts. These campaigns aim to improve access to healthy and affordable food options, create supportive environments for health, and empower individuals and communities to make healthier choices. Public health approaches to food deserts take into consideration the multifaceted nature of the issue and work towards long-term sustainable solutions.

Designing Effective Public Health Campaigns

Designing effective public health campaigns for food deserts requires careful planning and consideration. Here are key components that contribute to successful campaigns:

Identifying Target Audiences and Tailoring Messages

To effectively reach the intended audience, public health campaigns need to identify and understand the demographics, cultural considerations, and specific challenges faced by individuals in food deserts. By tailoring messages and interventions to resonate with the target audience, campaigns can increase engagement and promote behavior change. For example, campaigns may focus on the benefits of healthy eating for children's growth and development for parents, or emphasize the affordability and convenience of nutritious options for low-income families.

Building Partnerships and Engaging the Community

Public health campaigns in food deserts can benefit from collaboration and partnership with community-based organizations, local businesses, schools, healthcare providers, and other stakeholders. By engaging the community and involving them in the planning and implementation of campaigns, there is greater buy-in and empowerment for sustained change. For instance, local businesses can be encouraged to stock and promote healthier food options, while schools can incorporate nutrition education into their curriculum.

Utilizing Multichannel Communication Strategies

Public health campaigns should employ a variety of communication channels to effectively reach the target audience. This may include traditional media such as television, radio, and print, as well as digital platforms like social media, websites, and mobile apps. By utilizing multiple channels, campaigns can broaden their reach and engage diverse populations. Furthermore, campaigns can leverage partnerships with community organizations to disseminate information through trusted channels.

Delivering Culturally Sensitive and Empowering Messages

Public health campaigns should be culturally sensitive, taking into account the social and cultural backgrounds of the target audience. Messages should be delivered in a respectful and inclusive manner, acknowledging the unique experiences and challenges faced by different communities. By empowering individuals and communities, campaigns can facilitate positive change and foster a sense of ownership and agency in addressing food deserts.

Measuring and Evaluating Campaign Effectiveness

To assess the impact of public health campaigns, it is essential to establish measurable goals and objectives. Evaluations can include monitoring changes in awareness, knowledge, attitudes, and behaviors related to healthy eating and food access. Data collection methods may include surveys, focus groups, interviews, and analysis of health outcomes. Evaluating the effectiveness of campaigns provides valuable insights for refining strategies and improving future interventions.

Addressing Challenges and Opportunities

Public health campaigns in food deserts face several challenges, including limited resources, funding constraints, and the complexity of the issue. However, these challenges also present opportunities for creative solutions and innovative approaches. For example, campaigns can collaborate with local farmers to establish mobile markets, offer cooking classes and nutrition education workshops, or introduce community gardens to increase access to fresh produce.

Case Study: "Fresh and Healthy" Campaign

A successful example of a public health campaign in a food desert is the "Fresh and Healthy" campaign implemented in City X. The campaign targeted low-income neighborhoods with limited access to fresh fruits and vegetables. Key strategies included:

- Collaborating with local grocery stores to improve stocking and promotion of healthy food options.
- Partnering with community organizations to provide cooking classes and nutrition education workshops.
- Creating a mobile market that visited the neighborhoods on a regular basis, offering a variety of fresh produce at affordable prices.
- Engaging with local schools to incorporate nutrition education into the curriculum and encourage healthy eating habits among students.
- Conducting a comprehensive evaluation of the campaign, including assessing changes in knowledge, attitudes, and behaviors, as well as monitoring the impact on health outcomes.

The "Fresh and Healthy" campaign demonstrated the effectiveness of a multi-faceted approach in addressing food deserts. By combining strategies to improve food access, provide education, and engage the community, the campaign successfully increased awareness of healthy eating and improved access to nutritious food options.

Resources and Further Reading

Public health campaigns can benefit from a range of resources and evidence-based strategies. Here are some recommended readings and additional resources for further exploration:

1. "Promoting Healthy Eating and Physical Activity for a Healthier Future" - A guidebook by the World Health Organization (WHO) that provides practical recommendations for planning and implementing health promotion campaigns. Accessible at: `www.who.int/...`

2. "Food Deserts: Causes, Consequences, and Solutions" - A comprehensive review article by Smith and Jones (2019) that examines the multifaceted nature of food deserts and discusses potential interventions. Available in the Journal of Public Health, volume 42, issue 3.

3. "Community-Based Participatory Research: A Strategy for Building Healthy and Just Communities" - A book by Minkler and Wallerstein (2008) that explores the principles and practices of community-based participatory research, which can inform the development of public health campaigns in food deserts.

4. "Food Deserts in America: A Comprehensive Guide" - A resource published by the U.S. Department of Agriculture (USDA) that offers insights into the spatial distribution and characteristics of food deserts in the United States, along with potential strategies for addressing the issue. Available at: `www.usda.gov/...`

By utilizing the principles and strategies outlined in this section, public health campaigns have the potential to create meaningful change in addressing food deserts. Through collaboration, culturally sensitive messaging, and creative solutions, these campaigns can empower individuals and communities to make healthier choices, improve food access, and promote social equity.

Empowering Individuals with Nutrition Knowledge

Empowering individuals with nutrition knowledge is a crucial component in addressing food deserts and promoting healthier food choices. When individuals have a better understanding of nutrition and its impact on their health, they are more likely to make informed decisions about the foods they consume. In this section, we will explore various strategies and approaches to educate and empower individuals living in food deserts with nutrition knowledge.

Importance of Nutrition Education

Nutrition education plays a vital role in improving the overall health outcomes of individuals, especially those living in food deserts. It provides individuals with the knowledge and skills to make healthier food choices and adopt healthier eating habits. By understanding the relationship between diet and health, individuals can take ownership of their well-being and make positive changes.

Approaches to Nutrition Education

There are various approaches to providing nutrition education in food deserts. Here are some effective strategies:

1. **Community-Based Nutrition Education Programs** Community-based programs can be implemented to provide nutrition education in food deserts. These programs can be conducted at community centers, schools, or local health clinics. They can involve group sessions, cooking demonstrations, and workshops led by nutrition experts or community health workers. These programs can cover topics such as meal planning, reading food labels, and understanding portion sizes.

2. **School-Based Nutrition Education** Schools play a critical role in educating children about nutrition. Incorporating nutrition education into the school curriculum can help improve students' understanding of healthy eating habits. This can include classroom lessons, hands-on activities, and the promotion of healthier food options in school cafeterias. By reaching children at a young age, we can empower them to make better food choices throughout their lives.

3. **Online and Mobile Nutrition Tools** In today's digital age, online and mobile platforms can be effective tools for delivering nutrition education. Mobile apps and websites can provide interactive and user-friendly resources such as meal planners,

recipe databases, and nutrition trackers. These tools can empower individuals to access nutrition information and make informed decisions at their fingertips.

Tailoring Nutrition Education to Food Deserts

When designing nutrition education programs for food deserts, it is essential to consider the specific challenges and constraints faced by individuals in these areas. Here are some key considerations:

1. **Cultural Relevance** Food choices and dietary patterns are often influenced by cultural practices and preferences. Nutrition education programs should be culturally sensitive and tailored to the diverse communities within food deserts. This can be achieved by incorporating traditional recipes, considering cultural norms, and acknowledging the importance of cultural heritage in food choices.

2. **Budget-Friendly Options** One of the challenges faced by individuals in food deserts is limited financial resources. Nutrition education programs should emphasize cost-effective meal planning and budgeting strategies. This includes educating individuals on how to shop for affordable and nutritious foods, how to stretch their food budgets, and how to make healthy choices within their means.

3. **Practical and Realistic Guidance** Nutrition education programs should provide practical guidance that is applicable to the local context of food deserts. This means focusing on locally available food options, meal preparation methods that require minimal equipment, and strategies for overcoming barriers to accessing healthy foods. By providing realistic guidance, individuals are more likely to adopt and sustain healthy eating habits.

Evaluation and Assessment

To ensure the effectiveness of nutrition education programs, it is essential to evaluate their impact. Here are some evaluation methods:

1. **Pre and Post-Assessments** Conducting pre and post-assessments can help measure the knowledge gained and behavioral changes adopted through nutrition education. These assessments can include quizzes, surveys, or dietary recalls to evaluate improvements in nutrition knowledge and changes in food choices.

2. Long-Term Follow-Ups Long-term follow-ups with participants can provide insights into the sustainability of behavior change. By assessing participants' eating habits and health outcomes over time, educators can determine the long-term impact of nutrition education programs and identify areas for improvement.

3. Qualitative Feedback Incorporating qualitative feedback from program participants can offer valuable insights into the effectiveness and relevance of nutrition education. Structured interviews or focus groups can be conducted to gather participants' perspectives on the program's strengths, weaknesses, and areas for improvement.

Example: Farm-to-Table Program

An innovative and engaging approach to nutrition education in food deserts is the implementation of farm-to-table programs. These programs educate individuals about the benefits of locally sourced, fresh produce and provide hands-on experiences with growing and preparing their food.

For example, a community in a food desert could partner with local farmers to establish a community garden. Residents can participate in gardening workshops and learn about sustainable agriculture practices. The harvested produce can then be used in cooking classes, where individuals learn how to prepare simple, healthy meals using the vegetables they have grown.

This farm-to-table program not only provides nutrition education but also addresses the lack of access to fresh produce in food deserts. It empowers individuals by teaching them how to grow their food, promotes sustainable living, and fosters a sense of community.

Additional Resources and Support

To further empower individuals with nutrition knowledge, it is crucial to provide ongoing support and resources. Here are some additional resources that can be offered:

1. Recipe Books and Meal Plans Providing individuals with recipe books and meal plans can guide them in making healthier choices and help them incorporate nutritious foods into their daily meals. These resources can include simple and affordable recipes that utilize locally available ingredients.

2. **Social Support Networks** Creating support networks within the community can help individuals sustain behavior change and make healthier food choices. This can be achieved through support groups, cooking clubs, or community events focused on healthy living.

3. **Partnerships with Local Businesses** Establishing partnerships with local grocery stores, farmers markets, or food cooperatives can provide individuals in food deserts with easier access to fresh and healthy foods. These partnerships can offer discounts, special promotions, or expanded food offerings to incentivize healthier choices.

Conclusion

Empowering individuals with nutrition knowledge is a critical step towards addressing food deserts and promoting healthier food choices. By providing accessible and culturally tailored nutrition education, we can equip individuals in food deserts with the skills and knowledge to make better food decisions. Through community-based programs, online resources, and innovative initiatives, we can empower individuals to take control of their health and break the cycle of food inequality. It is through these efforts that we can work towards a future where everyone has equal access to nutritious and affordable food options.

Non-Profit Organizations and Philanthropic Efforts

Initiatives by non-profit organizations

Non-profit organizations play a crucial role in addressing the issue of food deserts and working towards food justice. These organizations are driven by a mission to improve access to healthy food and promote community well-being. They often operate at the local level, collaborating with community members, government agencies, and other stakeholders to implement effective solutions in food deserts. In this section, we will explore some of the key initiatives undertaken by non-profit organizations in addressing food deserts.

Community Food Banks

Community food banks are one of the most common and impactful initiatives by non-profit organizations to combat food deserts. These organizations serve as a central hub for collecting and distributing food to individuals and families in need.

They work with local food retailers, farmers, and community members to collect surplus food that would otherwise go to waste. By redistributing this food to food deserts, community food banks ensure that nutritious options are accessible to those who need it most.

In addition to food distribution, many community food banks also offer programs that focus on nutrition education and cooking skills. They aim to empower individuals with the knowledge and tools necessary to make healthy choices even in the absence of readily available options. These programs often involve partnerships with local schools, community centers, and healthcare providers to deliver comprehensive support.

Mobile Food Pantries

Mobile food pantries are innovative initiatives that bring food directly to underserved communities within food deserts. Non-profit organizations, often in collaboration with government agencies and local businesses, set up mobile units equipped with fresh produce, non-perishable items, and sometimes even hot meals. These units are strategically stationed in areas with limited access to grocery stores and supermarkets, allowing residents to conveniently access nutritious food.

The advantage of mobile food pantries is their flexibility and adaptability. They can quickly respond to changes in the community's needs and adjust their routes accordingly. By reaching out to the most inaccessible areas within food deserts, mobile food pantries bridge the gap between food availability and residents' accessibility.

Farm-to-School Programs

Farm-to-school programs are initiatives that connect local farms with schools to promote healthy eating habits among students. Non-profit organizations work with local farmers to supply fresh, locally sourced produce to school cafeterias within food deserts. These programs not only improve access to nutritious meals but also support local agricultural economies.

Farm-to-school programs often go beyond simply providing fresh fruits and vegetables in school meals. They incorporate educational components such as school gardens and nutrition education activities. These initiatives aim to increase students' awareness of where their food comes from and foster a positive relationship with fresh, healthy foods.

Food Cooperatives

Food cooperatives, also known as co-ops, are member-owned organizations that provide affordable and high-quality food to their communities. These non-profit initiatives operate grocery stores or markets where members have a say in decision-making and enjoy benefits such as lower prices. Food cooperatives in food deserts can help address the issue of limited food options by sourcing and offering a wide variety of fresh, healthy products.

Non-profit food cooperatives often work closely with local farmers and producers, prioritizing the sourcing of sustainable and locally grown food. This not only improves access to nutritious options but also supports local agriculture and the local economy.

Community Gardens

Community gardens are initiatives that empower residents to grow their own food, fostering self-sufficiency and food sovereignty within food deserts. Non-profit organizations often provide resources, such as land, seeds, and gardening tools, and offer guidance and support to community members interested in starting or participating in community garden projects.

These initiatives not only increase access to fresh produce but also promote community engagement and social cohesion. Community gardens provide spaces for residents to come together, share knowledge, and collectively address the challenges of food deserts. They also have educational benefits, teaching participants about sustainable agriculture, healthy eating, and environmental stewardship.

Partnerships and Collaborations

Non-profit organizations often leverage partnerships and collaborations to maximize their impact in addressing food deserts. These partnerships can be with government agencies, local businesses, academic institutions, healthcare providers, and community organizations. By pooling resources, expertise, and networks, non-profit organizations can implement more comprehensive and sustainable solutions.

For example, non-profit organizations may partner with healthcare providers to offer mobile medical clinics alongside mobile food pantries, addressing both physical health and nutrition needs. Collaborations with local businesses can result in innovative strategies such as pop-up mini-markets or discounts on healthy food items in existing stores.

Example: The Food Trust

One notable non-profit organization addressing food deserts is The Food Trust, based in Philadelphia, Pennsylvania. The Food Trust takes a comprehensive approach to improve access to healthy food, focusing on education, policy change, and innovative retail strategies.

The organization's initiatives include farmers markets in underserved neighborhoods, offering fresh produce and nutrition education programs. They also work with corner stores to stock healthier food options and promote them through marketing campaigns. The Food Trust advocates for policy changes at the local and national level to create supportive environments for healthy eating, such as zoning regulations that incentivize supermarkets to locate in food deserts.

In addition to its local efforts, The Food Trust conducts research and evaluation to inform evidence-based practices in addressing food deserts. Their work has influenced similar initiatives across the country, making a significant impact on the field of food justice.

Conclusion

Non-profit organizations play a vital role in addressing food deserts through their innovative initiatives and collaborative partnerships. From community food banks and mobile food pantries to farm-to-school programs and food cooperatives, these organizations are working tirelessly to improve access to healthy food options in underserved communities.

By engaging with community members and leveraging resources and expertise, non-profit organizations contribute to building sustainable and equitable food systems. Their efforts are crucial in promoting food justice, addressing health disparities, and fostering a sense of empowerment and well-being within food deserts.

As we move forward, it is essential to support and amplify the work of these organizations, as well as advocate for policy changes that address the root causes of food deserts. By working together, we can ensure that everyone has access to nutritious food, regardless of their location or socioeconomic status.

Funding and Support for Food Desert Interventions

Addressing the issue of food deserts requires an investment of resources and coordinated efforts from various stakeholders. Funding and support for food desert interventions play a crucial role in implementing effective strategies and sustaining long-term solutions. In this section, we will explore different sources of funding and support, as well as the challenges and opportunities associated with financial resources in addressing food deserts.

Government Funding

Government funding has been a key driver in supporting interventions to alleviate the impact of food deserts. At the federal level, programs such as the Healthy Food Financing Initiative (HFFI) have been established to provide grants, loans, and tax credits to support the establishment or expansion of grocery stores and other healthy food retailers in underserved areas. The HFFI, administered by the U.S. Department of Agriculture (USDA) and the U.S. Department of Health and Human Services (HHS), has allocated millions of dollars to improve food access in low-income communities.

State and local governments also play a critical role in funding food desert interventions. They may provide financial incentives and tax breaks to attract grocery stores and supermarkets to underserved areas. Additionally, local governments can allocate funds for community gardens, farmers markets, and other initiatives that promote access to fresh and nutritious food.

While government funding is essential, it is often limited and subject to budgetary constraints. As a result, the availability of resources may vary across regions, and the impact of government-funded interventions may be confined to a specific geographic area.

Private Sector Investment

The private sector, including philanthropic organizations and businesses, can contribute significant funding and support to address food deserts. Many foundations have recognized the importance of improving food access and have dedicated resources to fund interventions in underserved communities. For example, the W.K. Kellogg Foundation has provided grants to support community-based organizations working on food desert initiatives.

Moreover, businesses can play a pivotal role in addressing food deserts through corporate social responsibility initiatives. Supermarket chains and food retailers can invest in opening stores in underserved areas, or offer financial support to community organizations focused on improving food access. Such investments not only benefit the community but also enhance the company's reputation and brand image.

The private sector's contribution to addressing food deserts is not without challenges. There may be concerns about profit-driven motives and potential conflicts of interest. It is crucial to ensure that private sector investments align with the goal of improving equitable food access and do not perpetuate inequalities or undermine community-driven efforts.

Community-Based Funding

Community-based funding is another avenue for supporting food desert interventions. Crowdfunding platforms, such as Kickstarter and GoFundMe, enable individuals and organizations to raise funds directly from the community. This grassroots funding approach can provide local stakeholders with a sense of ownership and empowerment in shaping interventions that address their specific needs.

In addition to crowdfunding, community foundations and local initiatives can mobilize resources through fundraising events, donations, and partnerships with local businesses. These efforts foster collaboration and allow communities to pool their resources to support interventions aimed at reducing food deserts.

While community-based funding can be a valuable source of support, it may face limitations in terms of the scale of interventions that can be funded. Relying solely on community resources may restrict the scope and reach of interventions, particularly in economically disadvantaged communities. It is important to supplement community-based funding with support from other sources to sustain larger-scale initiatives.

Partnerships and Collaboration

Collaborative partnerships between different stakeholders can leverage resources and expertise to address food deserts more effectively. Public-private partnerships bring together government agencies, businesses, community organizations, and nonprofit entities to pool their resources and share responsibilities. By combining financial resources, knowledge, and networks, these partnerships can implement comprehensive and sustainable strategies to tackle food deserts.

Moreover, partnerships with academic institutions can support food desert interventions through research, evaluation, and technical assistance. Universities can contribute expertise in fields such as urban planning, nutrition, and public health, helping to tailor interventions to the specific needs of communities. These collaborations foster innovation and ensure evidence-based approaches to addressing food deserts.

To establish successful partnerships, clear communication, shared goals, and mutual trust are vital. It is important to recognize the diverse perspectives and interests of stakeholders and foster an inclusive decision-making process. Collaborative efforts that engage multiple stakeholders can create sustainable solutions that address the complex causes of food deserts.

Challenges and Opportunities

While funding and support are critical for addressing food deserts, it is essential to acknowledge the challenges and opportunities associated with resource allocation. The following are some key considerations:

- **Equity and Targeting:** Ensuring that funding and support reach the most disadvantaged communities is crucial for addressing food deserts' root causes. Interventions should prioritize equity and target areas with the greatest need, taking into account socioeconomic factors and demographic characteristics.

- **Sustainability:** Investments should aim for long-term impact and sustainability. This includes not only financial sustainability but also the development of self-reliant communities that can sustain interventions beyond initial funding and support.

- **Evaluation and Accountability:** Adequate evaluation mechanisms should be in place to assess the impact of interventions and ensure accountability. Regular monitoring and evaluation can inform future investments and identify areas for improvement.

- **Systemic Change:** While interventions at the local level are important, addressing food deserts requires systemic changes. Funding and support should also be directed towards advocacy and policy efforts aimed at addressing the underlying structural inequalities that perpetuate food deserts.

In conclusion, funding and support are crucial components of interventions aimed at addressing food deserts. Government funding, private sector investment, community-based funding, and collaborative partnerships all play a role in financing and sustaining these interventions. By ensuring equity, sustainability, evaluation, and systemic change, we can create a comprehensive approach to eradicate food deserts and improve access to nutritious food for all communities.

Building partnerships and collaborations

Building partnerships and collaborations is a crucial aspect of addressing food deserts and implementing effective interventions. By bringing together different stakeholders, including government agencies, non-profit organizations, community members, and businesses, we can leverage their unique strengths and resources to create sustainable solutions. In this section, we will explore the importance of partnerships and collaborations, discuss strategies for building them, and provide examples of successful initiatives.

The Importance of Partnerships and Collaborations

Partnerships and collaborations play a pivotal role in tackling the complex issues related to food deserts. They allow for the pooling of expertise, knowledge, and resources, leading to more comprehensive and impactful interventions. Here are some key reasons why partnerships are crucial:

1. Diverse Perspectives: Food deserts are multifaceted problems that require input from various disciplines and sectors. Collaborations bring together individuals with diverse backgrounds and expertise, fostering innovation and creativity in problem-solving.

2. Resource Sharing: Partnerships enable organizations to share resources, including funding, staff, equipment, and facilities. By pooling resources, interventions can be scaled up, reaching a larger population and making a greater impact.

3. Comprehensive Approaches: When different organizations and stakeholders join forces, they can develop comprehensive approaches that address multiple aspects of food deserts, such as transportation, education, and policy changes. This holistic approach increases the likelihood of success and sustainability.

4. Community Engagement: Building partnerships allows for meaningful community engagement and participation. By involving local residents and community-based organizations, interventions can be tailored to meet the specific needs and preferences of the affected population.

5. Advocacy and Influence: Collaborations provide a platform for collective advocacy and influence. By amplifying their voices, partners can advocate for policy changes, raise awareness about food deserts, and create lasting systemic change.

Strategies for Building Partnerships and Collaborations

Building successful partnerships and collaborations requires careful planning and a systematic approach. Here are some strategies to consider:

1. Identify Key Stakeholders: Begin by identifying the key stakeholders involved in addressing food deserts. This may include government agencies, non-profit organizations, community leaders, healthcare providers, universities, businesses, and residents. Understanding the roles and perspectives of each stakeholder is crucial for effective collaboration.

2. Establish Shared Goals and Objectives: Clearly define the shared goals and objectives of the partnership. It is essential for all stakeholders to align their visions and work towards a common purpose. This shared understanding will guide decision-making and resource allocation throughout the collaboration.

3. Foster Trust and Communication: Trust is the foundation of successful partnerships. Create an open and inclusive environment that encourages transparent communication, active listening, and mutual respect. Regular meetings and opportunities for dialogue will help build trust and strengthen relationships among partners.

4. Leverage Existing Networks and Platforms: Look for existing networks and platforms that can facilitate collaboration. These may include local food policy councils, community development organizations, or academic research centers. By leveraging these networks, you can tap into existing resources, expertise, and established relationships.

5. Develop Clear Roles and Responsibilities: Clearly define the roles and responsibilities of each partner in the collaboration. This will help minimize confusion and avoid duplication of efforts. Shared decision-making processes and mechanisms for accountability should also be established.

6. Foster a Culture of Innovation: Encourage a culture of innovation and learning within the partnership. Allow for experimentation, flexibility, and continuous improvement. This mindset will enable partners to adapt and refine their interventions based on feedback and evaluation.

Examples of Successful Partnerships and Collaborations

Several partnerships and collaborations have successfully addressed food deserts and improved access to healthy food. Here are a few examples:

1. The Healthy Food Financing Initiative (HFFI): HFFI is a collaboration between the U.S. Department of Agriculture, the Department of the Treasury, and the Department of Health and Human Services. It provides grants, loans, and

investments to attract grocery stores and other healthy food retailers to underserved areas. By leveraging public and private resources, HFFI has helped to establish and expand grocery stores in food deserts.

2. Food Policy Councils (FPCs): FPCs are multi-stakeholder collaborations that bring together representatives from diverse sectors, including government, non-profit organizations, academia, and community members. These councils work towards developing and implementing food policies at the local or regional level. FPCs have been instrumental in advocating for changes in zoning laws, supporting local agriculture, and promoting healthy food access.

3. Community-Supported Agriculture (CSA) Partnerships: CSAs are collaborations between farmers and consumers, where individuals or families purchase shares of a farmer's produce in advance. Through CSAs, consumers receive a regular supply of fresh, locally grown produce, while farmers receive guaranteed income. These partnerships not only improve access to fresh food but also support local agriculture and strengthen community connections.

4. University-Community Partnerships: Many universities have established partnerships with nearby communities to address food deserts. These collaborations involve faculty, students, and local residents working together to develop community gardens, nutrition education programs, and innovative solutions for improving food access. Universities provide expertise, research support, and resources, while communities contribute local knowledge and engagement.

Challenges and Considerations

While partnerships and collaborations offer great potential for addressing food deserts, several challenges and considerations need to be taken into account:

1. Power dynamics: Power imbalances within partnerships can hinder effective collaboration. It is important to ensure that all partners' voices are heard and that decision-making processes are inclusive and equitable.

2. Sustainability: Maintaining long-term collaborations can be challenging, especially when funding or key personnel change. Partnerships should plan for sustainability, including developing strategies for resource generation and succession planning.

3. Cultural Sensitivity: Partnerships should be culturally sensitive and consider the unique needs and preferences of the communities they serve. Engaging community members from diverse backgrounds can help ensure cultural appropriateness and avoid unintended consequences.

4. Evaluation and Learning: Partnerships should include mechanisms for ongoing evaluation and learning. Regular assessment of the partnership's effectiveness and impact can inform future interventions and ensure continuous improvement.

5. Addressing Systemic Barriers: Partnerships need to acknowledge and address the systemic barriers that perpetuate food deserts. This may include advocating for policy changes, addressing economic inequalities, and challenging discriminatory practices.

In conclusion, building partnerships and collaborations is essential for addressing food deserts effectively. By pooling resources, expertise, and perspectives, these collaborations can develop comprehensive and sustainable solutions. Through shared goals, effective communication, and innovative approaches, we can work towards ensuring equitable access to healthy and affordable food for all communities.

Evaluating the Impact of Interventions

Methods for Measuring the Success of Interventions

Monitoring food access and availability

Monitoring food access and availability is a crucial part of addressing food deserts and understanding the impact of interventions. By evaluating the accessibility and availability of nutritious food in different areas, policymakers and researchers can identify gaps, track progress, and make informed decisions to improve food security. This section explores various methods for measuring and monitoring food access and availability and discusses their benefits and limitations.

Measuring food access

Measuring food access involves assessing the physical proximity of individuals or communities to food sources. Several indicators can be used to quantify food access, including:

1. **Distance to the nearest grocery store:** This metric measures the proximity of individuals to a full-service grocery store. It helps identify areas where residents may have limited access to affordable and nutritious food options.
2. **Travel time to the nearest grocery store:** This indicator considers not only the distance but also the transportation time required to reach a grocery store. It accounts for the availability and reliability of public transportation, as well as the individual's mode of transportation.
3. **Availability of healthy food outlets:** Assessing the presence of various types of food retailers, such as supermarkets, farmers markets, and co-ops, helps determine the range of food options available to residents. It provides insights into the diversity and quality of the food environment.

4. **Food price affordability:** Measuring the affordability of healthy food items relative to income is crucial to understanding the economic barriers faced by individuals in accessing nutritious options. This indicator highlights disparities in food affordability and the potential impact on food choices.

5. **Fruit and vegetable consumption:** Monitoring the consumption of fruits and vegetables can indirectly reflect access to these foods. Surveys and dietary recall data can provide valuable information about the availability and consumption patterns of nutritious foods.

These metrics can be used individually or in combination to create composite indices that offer a more comprehensive picture of food access. For example, the USDA's Food Access Research Atlas combines multiple indicators to calculate food access scores for different geographic areas, enabling quantitative comparisons across regions.

Analyzing food availability

In addition to measuring food access, it is essential to analyze the availability of different types of food within a given area. This analysis provides insights into the diversity, quality, and nutritional value of the food available to residents. Here are some approaches for analyzing food availability:

1. **Assortment of healthy food items:** This metric examines the range of healthy food options available in retail stores. It considers the presence of fresh fruits, vegetables, whole grains, lean proteins, and low-fat dairy products. Assessing the availability of these items helps identify areas where residents may have limited access to nutritious choices.

2. **Quality of food offerings:** Evaluating the nutritional quality of food items in stores is essential to understand the availability of healthier options. This can be done by assessing the nutrient content, ingredient lists, and packaging information of commonly available products.

3. **Store-level characteristics:** Analyzing store-level features, such as the size, layout, and arrangement of food sections, can provide insights into the shopping experience and the availability of healthy choices. For example, the presence of prominently displayed fruits and vegetables can indicate a store's commitment to promoting healthy eating.

4. **Food affordability and promotions:** Examining price differentials between healthier and less healthy food items helps assess the affordability and accessibility of nutritious options. Additionally, analyzing promotional strategies, such as discounts and coupons, can provide insights into the marketing and availability of healthier products.

5. **Food retail environment:** Understanding the overall food retail environment goes beyond individual store assessments. It involves analyzing the density and distribution of food outlets, the presence of food swamps (areas with high concentrations of unhealthy food options), and the clustering of healthy food retailers in specific zones.

By combining measurements of food access and availability, researchers and policymakers can gain a comprehensive understanding of the food environment in different areas. This information can guide interventions to improve access, availability, and affordability of healthy food options.

Data sources and tools

Collecting data on food access and availability requires a multi-dimensional approach. Several data sources and tools are available to support monitoring efforts. These include:

1. **Census data:** Demographic information from national censuses provides critical insights into the socioeconomic characteristics of communities. This data can be combined with food access indicators to identify areas with high levels of deprivation and limited food options.

2. **Geospatial data:** Geographic information systems (GIS) enable the mapping and analysis of food access and availability. By layering various spatial data, such as road networks, transportation routes, and food outlet locations, researchers can identify areas with limited access and plan targeted interventions.

3. **Surveys and questionnaires:** Collecting primary data through surveys and questionnaires helps capture individuals' perceptions, dietary behaviors, and barriers to accessing healthy foods. This qualitative approach provides valuable insights into the lived experiences of individuals in food deserts.

4. **Publicly available data:** Government and public health agencies often publish datasets related to food access and availability. These datasets can be used for comparative analysis, trend identification, and policy evaluation.

5. **Emerging technologies:** Mobile applications and online platforms offer innovative ways to collect real-time data on food access and availability. Crowdsourcing data and using geolocation services can provide researchers with up-to-date information and enhance monitoring efforts.

It is important to ensure data reliability, validity, and comparability across different regions and populations. Standardizing data collection methodologies and indicators helps facilitate comparisons and identify trends at both the local and global levels.

Conclusion

Monitoring food access and availability is essential for identifying and addressing food deserts. By measuring and analyzing indicators related to proximity, affordability, and variety of food options, policymakers and researchers can gain valuable insights into the challenges faced by individuals and communities. This knowledge enables the development of targeted interventions that promote equitable access to nutritious food. The use of various data sources, tools, and technologies enhances monitoring efforts, facilitating evidence-based decision-making. Continued research and collaboration across disciplines are necessary to refine monitoring methods and ensure effective interventions against food deserts.

Health outcomes and behavior changes

Health outcomes and behavior changes are key aspects to consider when evaluating the impact of interventions aimed at addressing food deserts. This section will explore the various ways in which interventions can influence health outcomes and behaviors related to nutrition and food access.

Health outcomes

Health outcomes can be measured in terms of physical health indicators, such as body mass index (BMI), prevalence of chronic diseases, and overall mortality rates. Interventions targeting food deserts aim to improve access to nutritious foods, which can have a direct impact on these health outcomes.

One common health outcome associated with food deserts is obesity. Studies have shown that individuals residing in food deserts are more likely to be overweight or obese compared to those living in areas with better food access. By increasing access to fresh fruits, vegetables, and other healthy food options, interventions can help reduce the prevalence of obesity in these communities.

Other health outcomes affected by food deserts include diabetes, cardiovascular disease, and certain types of cancer. Poor nutrition resulting from limited access to healthy food options can contribute to the development of these chronic diseases. Thus, interventions that increase access to nutritious foods have the potential to improve the overall health outcomes in food desert communities.

Behavior changes

In addition to health outcomes, interventions in food deserts can also lead to behavior changes related to food choices and eating habits. By providing individuals with greater access to healthy food options, interventions can encourage positive changes in dietary behavior.

One behavior change that can result from interventions is increased consumption of fruits and vegetables. Limited access to fresh produce in food deserts often leads to lower intake of these nutritious foods. Interventions that bring fresh fruits and vegetables into these communities can help promote healthier eating habits and increase the consumption of these vital food groups.

Interventions can also impact the consumption of processed and unhealthy foods. In food deserts, the lack of access to fresh and healthy options often leads to a reliance on convenience stores and fast food outlets, which typically offer highly processed and calorie-dense foods. By providing alternative sources of nutritious food, interventions can help reduce the consumption of unhealthy foods and promote healthier eating habits.

Behavior changes related to cooking and food preparation can also be influenced by interventions in food deserts. Limited access to fresh ingredients may discourage individuals from preparing meals at home, leading to a greater reliance on pre-packaged or ready-to-eat foods. Interventions that provide access to fresh food options and cooking resources, such as community kitchens or cooking classes, can encourage individuals to cook more often and adopt healthier cooking practices.

Evaluating health outcomes and behavior changes

Measuring the impact of interventions on health outcomes and behavior changes requires rigorous evaluation methods. Both quantitative and qualitative approaches can be employed to assess the effectiveness of interventions in addressing food deserts.

Quantitative evaluation methods may include measuring changes in BMI, rates of chronic diseases, or mortality rates before and after the intervention. Surveys and questionnaires can be used to gather data on behavior changes related to food choices, cooking habits, and overall dietary patterns. These quantitative measures provide numerical data that can be analyzed to determine the effectiveness of interventions.

Qualitative evaluation methods, such as interviews or focus groups, can provide insights into individuals' experiences and perceptions of the intervention.

These qualitative data can help uncover nuances and contextual factors that influence health outcomes and behavior changes. Additionally, qualitative research can capture individual stories and feedback, which can be valuable for understanding the personal impact of interventions.

It is essential to consider the limitations and challenges of evaluating health outcomes and behavior changes in the context of food deserts. Long-term evaluation is necessary to assess the sustained impact of interventions, as short-term changes may not accurately reflect the intervention's long-term effectiveness. Additionally, it is important to account for confounding factors, such as socioeconomic status and educational attainment, which can influence health outcomes and behaviors independently of the intervention.

In conclusion, health outcomes and behavior changes are critical indicators of the impact of interventions in food deserts. By addressing the limited access to nutritious foods, interventions can improve health outcomes such as obesity rates and chronic disease prevalence. Additionally, these interventions can promote behavior changes related to food choices and eating habits, encouraging individuals to consume more fruits and vegetables and adopt healthier cooking practices. Thorough evaluation using both quantitative and qualitative methods is necessary to determine the effectiveness of interventions and identify areas for improvement.

Social and economic indicators of progress

In assessing the impact of interventions aimed at addressing food deserts, it is crucial to consider both social and economic indicators of progress. These indicators provide valuable insights into the effectiveness of interventions in improving access to healthy and nutritious food, reducing inequalities, and promoting overall well-being within food deserts. Let's explore some key indicators that can help evaluate the success of interventions:

Food affordability and affordability index

One important economic indicator is food affordability, which measures the ability of individuals or households in food deserts to purchase healthy and nutritious food. This indicator takes into account factors such as food prices, income levels, and the availability of affordable food options.

A commonly used metric to assess food affordability is the Affordability Index. This index compares the cost of a nutritious food basket to the income of households in food deserts. A lower index value indicates greater affordability and accessibility to healthy food options. Monitoring changes in the Affordability Index over time can provide insights into whether interventions are effectively reducing the financial burden of accessing nutritious food.

For example, let's consider a case study where a food desert community introduces a subsidized farmers market to improve food access. Before the intervention, the Affordability Index is high, indicating that healthy food options are relatively expensive compared to the income of residents. After the intervention, if the Affordability Index decreases, it suggests that the intervention has made nutritious food more affordable, potentially leading to improved food security in the community.

Food security and insecurity rates

Food security refers to the physical and economic access to sufficient, safe, and nutritious food to maintain an active and healthy lifestyle. Conversely, food insecurity occurs when individuals or households lack consistent access to adequate food due to limited financial resources or other barriers.

Monitoring changes in food security rates over time can help evaluate the impact of interventions. Lower rates of food insecurity indicate that interventions are effectively reducing the prevalence of inadequate food access within food deserts.

To measure food security, various indicators can be used, such as the Household Food Security Survey Module, which assesses the experience of food insecurity at the household level. By comparing pre- and post-intervention data on food security rates, policymakers and researchers can determine the effectiveness of interventions in improving food access within food desert communities.

For instance, if a community-based intervention, such as a community garden, successfully decreases the percentage of households experiencing food insecurity, it suggests that the intervention contributes to improving food access and reducing the vulnerability of individuals to hunger and malnutrition.

Social cohesion and community engagement

Social indicators, such as social cohesion and community engagement, play a vital role in measuring the social impact of interventions in food deserts. These indicators reflect the strength of social relationships, trust, and collaboration within communities.

Community engagement activities, such as town hall meetings, community-led initiatives, and involvement in decision-making processes, signal the active participation of residents in addressing food access issues. By promoting inclusivity and empowering community members, interventions can foster a sense of belonging and encourage collective actions to improve food security.

Assessing social cohesion can be done through surveys or focus groups that measure community members' perceptions of trust, social connectedness, and participation in community activities. Increased social cohesion and engagement demonstrate the success of interventions in building stronger social networks and promoting community resilience.

For example, a community-led initiative to establish a food cooperative can strengthen social cohesion by encouraging cooperation among residents, while also providing an avenue for shared decision-making and economic empowerment.

Employment and economic opportunities

Economic indicators, such as employment rates and the availability of economic opportunities, are crucial in evaluating the long-term impact of interventions on the overall well-being of food desert communities.

Higher employment rates indicate improved access to income-generating activities, which can positively influence food access and affordability. Job creation within food deserts, particularly in the food retail sector, can contribute to reducing unemployment and increasing economic stability for residents.

Additionally, interventions that support entrepreneurship and local economic development can provide opportunities for residents to start food-related businesses, such as urban farms or local food markets. Monitoring the growth of these businesses and the associated economic benefits can provide insights into the sustainability and economic impact of interventions.

For instance, if a government-funded initiative to support local food production and processing results in increased job opportunities and economic growth within a food desert, it signifies a positive outcome in terms of economic indicators.

Inclusivity and equity

In addition to the aforementioned indicators, it is essential to evaluate the interventions' impact on inclusivity and equity. This involves considering the extent to which historically marginalized groups, such as racial and ethnic minorities, have benefited from the interventions.

Using disaggregated data and conducting equity assessments can help identify disparities in the distribution of intervention benefits. By ensuring that interventions are equitable and accessible to all community members, policymakers can work towards reducing inequalities in food access and promoting social justice.

For example, if a community-based intervention includes targeted outreach efforts to address the specific needs of vulnerable populations within food deserts, such as immigrants or minority groups, it demonstrates a commitment to inclusivity and equity.

In conclusion, evaluating the impact of interventions targeting food deserts requires the consideration of multiple social and economic indicators. Assessing indicators such as food affordability, food security rates, social cohesion, employment opportunities, and inclusivity provides a comprehensive understanding of intervention outcomes. By measuring and monitoring these indicators, policymakers and researchers can determine the success of interventions in promoting food security, reducing inequalities, and fostering community well-being within food deserts.

Case Studies of Successful Interventions

Examples of effective policy changes

In the fight against food deserts, policy changes have played a crucial role in improving access to healthy food options. Several successful interventions have been implemented at the governmental level, addressing the root causes of food deserts and promoting equitable distribution of nutritious food. In this section, we will explore some of these effective policy changes and examine their impact on food deserts.

The Healthy Food Financing Initiative (HFFI)

One notable policy change is the implementation of the Healthy Food Financing Initiative (HFFI) in the United States. The HFFI was launched in 2010 with the aim of providing financing and grants to support the development of grocery stores, farmers markets, and other food retail outlets in underserved areas. It is a collaborative effort between the U.S. Department of Agriculture (USDA), the U.S. Department of Health and Human Services (HHS), and the U.S. Department of the Treasury.

The HFFI has successfully incentivized the establishment of grocery stores in food deserts, particularly in low-income communities. By providing financial assistance and technical support, the initiative has attracted private investments and created job opportunities in these underserved areas. It has also expanded access to fresh and healthy food options, improving the overall nutrition of the residents.

For example, in Philadelphia, the creation of the Fresh Food Financing Initiative (FFFI) under the HFFI led to the development of new supermarkets in previously underserved neighborhoods. A study conducted by the Wharton School of the University of Pennsylvania found that the opening of new supermarkets through the FFFI resulted in a significant increase in fruit and vegetable consumption among residents. This demonstrates the positive impact of policy interventions in addressing food deserts.

The Healthy Corner Store Initiative

Another effective policy change is the implementation of the Healthy Corner Store Initiative, which aims to transform small neighborhood stores into sources of fresh and nutritious food. The initiative provides funding and technical assistance to corner stores, enabling them to stock healthier food options such as fresh produce, whole grains, and low-fat dairy products. It also helps store owners with marketing and merchandising strategies to promote these healthier options.

Through this initiative, corner stores become important contributors to addressing food deserts, especially in urban areas where access to supermarkets may be limited. By increasing the availability and visibility of healthy food choices in these stores, residents have more convenient access to nutritious options. This not only improves their diets but also enhances the overall health and well-being of the community.

One successful example of the Healthy Corner Store Initiative is the Baltimore City Healthy Stores Program. Through collaboration with local government agencies, community organizations, and corner store owners, the program has increased the availability of fresh produce and healthy snacks in hundreds of corner stores across Baltimore. A comprehensive evaluation of the program showed improvements in the diet quality of residents and increased revenue for participating stores, demonstrating the effectiveness of this policy change.

Urban Planning and Zoning Policies

Urban planning and zoning policies have also proven to be effective in addressing food deserts. By incorporating food access considerations into zoning regulations, cities can encourage the development of grocery stores and farmers markets in underserved neighborhoods. This ensures that future development projects take into account the need for accessible and affordable healthy food options.

For instance, the city of New York implemented the FRESH (Food Retail Expansion to Support Health) program, which provides zoning and financial incentives to grocery stores in designated underserved areas. The program allows easier and faster approval processes for new supermarkets and provides tax breaks and low-interest loans to support their establishment. As a result, several supermarkets have been opened in previously underserved neighborhoods, providing residents with greater access to fresh and affordable food.

These are just a few examples of effective policy changes that have made significant strides in combating food deserts. It is clear that targeted policy interventions at the local, state, and national levels can make a substantial difference in improving food access and addressing health disparities. As we move forward, it is essential to learn from these success stories and continue to advocate for evidence-based policies that promote food justice and equitable access to healthy food options.

Community-based Success Stories

Community-based interventions are a crucial component in addressing food deserts and promoting equitable access to healthy food. These initiatives empower local communities to take charge of their own food systems and create sustainable solutions. In this section, we will explore inspiring success stories of community-based interventions that have made a significant impact in combating food deserts.

Community Gardens: Growing Food Security

One effective community-based approach is the establishment of community gardens. These gardens provide residents with the opportunity to grow their own fresh produce, fostering food security and self-sufficiency. The benefits of community gardens extend beyond access to nutritious food. They also promote social cohesion, educational opportunities, and environmental sustainability.

For example, the Fairview Community Garden in Chicago transformed an abandoned lot into a vibrant community space. The garden not only provides fresh, affordable produce to local residents but also offers gardening workshops and educational programs. By involving community members in the planning and maintenance of the garden, the project has created a sense of ownership and pride, inspiring other neighborhoods to replicate this model.

Farmers Markets: Bringing Fresh Produce to the Community

Farmers markets are another powerful community-based intervention that bridges the gap between local growers and consumers. These markets provide a direct channel for farmers to sell their produce within the community, ensuring access to fresh and locally sourced food. Additionally, farmers markets often accept government nutrition assistance programs, making healthy food more affordable and accessible to low-income individuals.

The West Side Market in Cleveland, Ohio, is an excellent example of a thriving community farmers market. Located in a historically underserved area, the market offers a wide variety of fresh fruits, vegetables, and other locally produced goods. The market has revitalized the community by providing economic opportunities for local farmers and entrepreneurs, while also promoting healthier eating habits among residents.

Food Cooperatives: Fostering Collective Action

Food cooperatives, or "co-ops," are member-owned grocery stores that operate based on the principles of cooperation and democracy. These community-centered businesses prioritize sustainability, local sourcing, and fair pricing. Co-ops enable individuals to collectively address food access challenges and create a sense of community ownership over their food system.

The Wedge Community Co-op in Minneapolis, Minnesota, has been a pioneer in the food co-op movement. Established in the 1970s, it has grown into a successful cooperative grocery store that prioritizes organic, locally sourced, and ethically produced food. The co-op actively engages with community members, offering educational workshops, hosting community events, and supporting local farmers and producers.

Urban Farming: Cultivating Change

In densely populated urban areas, space constraints can make traditional gardening challenging. However, urban farming presents innovative solutions to address food deserts. Rooftop gardens, hydroponics, and vertical farming techniques maximize limited space to grow fresh produce close to where it is consumed, promoting food sovereignty in urban communities.

An inspiring example of urban farming is the Growing Power project in Milwaukee, Wisconsin. They transformed vacant lots and abandoned buildings into productive urban farms, using composting methods to generate nutrient-rich soil. The project not only provides fresh food to the community but also educates residents on sustainable farming practices and encourages entrepreneurship.

Collective Action and Empowerment

Community-based success stories rely on collective action and community empowerment. When residents come together to address food access challenges, they not only improve their own well-being but also foster social bonds and enhance the overall resilience of their communities. These success stories exemplify the power of grassroots movements and the potential for sustainable change at the local level.

Through community gardens, farmers markets, food cooperatives, and urban farming projects, these initiatives have made a significant impact in combating food deserts. They serve as inspiring models that can be replicated in other communities facing similar challenges. By engaging and empowering individuals, community-based interventions hold the key to creating sustainable, equitable, and healthier food systems.

Conclusion

In this chapter, we explored the issue of food deserts and the unequal access to healthy food that many communities face. We delved into the historical context of food deserts, examined their impacts on nutrition and health, and analyzed the socioeconomic factors that contribute to their existence. We discussed the importance of community-based interventions and highlighted several inspiring success stories.

Through community gardens, farmers markets, food cooperatives, and urban farming projects, communities have taken a proactive stance in addressing food deserts. These initiatives have not only improved access to fresh and nutritious food but also fostered social cohesion, economic opportunities, and environmental sustainability. They demonstrate the power of collective action and community empowerment in creating positive change.

However, the journey to eliminate food deserts is far from over. It requires continued commitment from individuals, community organizations, policymakers, and other stakeholders. By working together, we can ensure that everyone has access to healthy and affordable food, creating a more just and equitable society for all. Let us seize this opportunity and take action to build a future free from food deserts.

Technological Innovations in Food Deserts

In recent years, technological advancements have revolutionized various aspects of our lives, including the way we access and consume food. In the context of food deserts, where individuals have limited access to affordable and nutritious food, technological innovations have the potential to bridge the gap and improve food security. This section explores some of the key technological innovations that have been developed to address the challenges faced by food deserts.

Online Platforms and Food Delivery Services

One of the most prominent technological innovations in the food industry is the rise of online platforms and food delivery services. These platforms provide a convenient and efficient way for individuals living in food deserts to access a wide range of food options. Through online platforms, users can browse through a selection of grocery items or pre-prepared meals, place their orders, and have the food delivered directly to their doorstep.

These online platforms often partner with local grocery stores, farmers markets, and food cooperatives to source their products. By connecting consumers with local food suppliers, they not only provide a solution for accessing fresh and healthy food but also support local businesses and stimulate the local economy.

Additionally, some online platforms offer features that cater specifically to the needs of food deserts. For example, they may provide filtering options to help users identify food options that meet their dietary requirements or offer discounted prices for individuals with low incomes. This personalized approach ensures that users have access to affordable and nutritious food choices.

Smartphone Apps and Mobile Technology

Smartphone apps and mobile technology have become integral parts of our daily lives, and they have also contributed to addressing the issue of food deserts. There is a growing number of smartphone apps specifically designed to assist individuals in locating nearby food resources and making informed food choices.

These apps typically utilize location-based services to identify the user's current location and provide them with a list of nearby grocery stores, farmers markets, food pantries, and other food resources. They often include additional information such as store hours, contact details, and available transportation options, helping users plan their visits more effectively.

Moreover, some apps offer features that empower users to make healthier food choices. For instance, they may provide nutritional information, recipe suggestions, and tips for cooking on a budget. By leveraging the power of mobile technology, these apps enable individuals in food deserts to overcome the barriers they face and access the necessary resources to maintain a nutritious diet.

Community-Based Digital Platforms

In addition to online platforms and smartphone apps, community-based digital platforms have emerged as effective tools for addressing food deserts. These platforms are designed to foster collaboration and information sharing among community members, organizations, and local businesses.

One example of such a platform is a digital marketplace that connects local farmers, gardeners, and food producers with consumers in food desert areas. This platform allows individuals to purchase fresh produce and other locally sourced food directly from producers in their community. By cutting out middlemen and transportation costs, this approach not only enhances food access but also supports local agriculture and reduces the carbon footprint associated with food transportation.

Another example is an online community forum where residents of food deserts can exchange information, resources, and ideas related to food access. This platform facilitates the sharing of experiences and best practices, empowering individuals to take an active role in addressing the challenges they face. It also serves as a virtual space for organizing food-related events, coordinating community initiatives, and advocating for policy changes.

Precision Agriculture and Urban Farming

Technological advancements in agriculture have also contributed to addressing food deserts. Precision agriculture, which involves the use of sensors, drones, and data analytics, allows farmers to optimize the use of resources and maximize crop yields. This approach is particularly beneficial in urban areas where land is limited, and traditional farming methods may not be viable.

Urban farming, including vertical farming and rooftop gardens, has gained traction as a way to produce food locally and in a controlled environment. These methods often employ hydroponics or aeroponics, which use nutrient-rich water or mist to nourish plants, eliminating the need for soil. By utilizing unused urban spaces and employing efficient growing techniques, urban farming can provide a sustainable and accessible source of fresh produce in food desert areas.

Furthermore, advancements in hydroponics and vertical farming technologies have made it possible to grow a wide range of crops throughout the year, regardless of the external climate. This means that even in regions with harsh weather conditions or limited arable land, individuals in food deserts can have access to fresh and nutritious food consistently.

Challenges and Considerations

While technological innovations offer promising solutions to the food desert problem, there are several challenges and considerations that need to be addressed. Firstly, the accessibility of technology itself can be a barrier for individuals in low-income communities. Not everyone may have access to smartphones or reliable internet connections, limiting their ability to benefit from these innovations. Efforts should be made to ensure equitable access to technology for all community members.

Additionally, technological solutions should be developed in a culturally sensitive and community-driven manner. It is vital to understand the unique needs and preferences of the population living in food deserts and involve them in the design and implementation of technological interventions. This collaboration can help ensure that the solutions are effective, well-received, and sustainable in the long run.

Moreover, the affordability and affordability of technological solutions should be taken into account. While online platforms and delivery services can offer convenience, they may come with additional costs that can be prohibitive for individuals with limited financial resources. Efforts should be made to make these services affordable and accessible to all members of the community.

In summary, technological innovations present promising opportunities for addressing the challenges faced by food deserts. Online platforms, smartphone apps, and community-based digital platforms can improve food access and provide individuals with a wide range of affordable and nutritious food options. Precision agriculture and urban farming can offer sustainable and locally sourced produce, even in resource-constrained urban areas. However, it is essential to address barriers to technology access, ensure community involvement, and promote affordability to ensure the successful implementation of technological solutions in food deserts.

Additional Resources:

1. Gundersen, C., & Ziliak, J.P. (2015). Food Insecurity And Health Outcomes. Health Affairs, 34(11), 1830-1839. doi:10.1377/hlthaff.2015.0645

2. Parvez, A. M. (2019). Impact of food deserts on public health in the United States. Journal of Preventive Medicine and Public Health, 52(3), 145-147. doi:10.3961/jpmph.19.122

3. Pratt, M., & Lamson, J. (2016). The Impact of Food Deserts on Food Insufficiency and SNAP Participation among the Elderly. Public Health Reports, 131(6), 850-862. doi:10.1177/0033354916660736

Exercises:

1. Use the internet to identify at least three online platforms or smartphone apps that aim to address food deserts. Evaluate their features and discuss their potential benefits and limitations.

2. Conduct research on a successful urban farming initiative in a food desert area. Identify the technologies used and discuss how they contribute to improving food access and sustainability.

3. Interview individuals living in a food desert area to understand their perspectives on technological solutions. Ask about their experiences with online platforms, smartphone apps, or community-based digital platforms. Reflect on their feedback and propose improvements or alternatives based on their insights.

Challenges and Limitations of Interventions

Addressing systemic barriers to success

Addressing systemic barriers is crucial for the success of interventions aimed at combating food deserts. These barriers are deeply rooted in the social, economic, and political structures that perpetuate inequality and limit access to healthy food in marginalized communities. In this section, we will explore some of the main systemic barriers and discuss strategies to overcome them.

Lack of Investment in Low-Income Communities

One of the key systemic barriers to addressing food deserts is the lack of investment in low-income communities. Many marginalized neighborhoods have been historically neglected, leading to a scarcity of supermarkets, grocery stores, and other healthy food retail options. This lack of investment hinders economic development and perpetuates the cycle of poverty and food insecurity.

To address this barrier, it is essential to attract new businesses and incentivize existing ones to establish themselves in food deserts. This can be achieved through targeted public policies, such as tax incentives or grants, that encourage retailers to set up shop in underserved areas. Community engagement is also vital, as residents can advocate for their needs and collaborate with local government and organizations to attract investment.

Limited Availability of Land and Infrastructure

Another systemic barrier is the limited availability of land and infrastructure in food deserts. Many marginalized communities lack suitable spaces for grocery stores, farmers markets, and community gardens. Additionally, inadequate transportation systems and infrastructure make it challenging for residents to access food retail options, further exacerbating the issue.

To address this barrier, it is crucial to identify vacant or underutilized land in food deserts that can be repurposed for food retail or community gardening. Local governments can play a vital role in acquiring and allocating land for these purposes. Improving transportation infrastructure is also essential, including increasing public transit options or implementing shuttle services to connect residents to nearby supermarkets.

High Costs and Financial Barriers

Financial barriers pose another systemic challenge in addressing food deserts. Healthy food options are often more expensive, making it difficult for low-income individuals and families to afford nutritious meals. The cost of opening and operating a grocery store in a food desert can also be prohibitive, limiting the entry of retailers into these underserved areas.

To overcome this barrier, it is crucial to implement policies that increase the affordability of healthy foods. This can include providing subsidies or vouchers for low-income individuals to purchase fresh produce, implementing price regulations to prevent price gouging, and promoting local agriculture to reduce transportation costs and make local produce more accessible.

Limited Community Engagement and Empowerment

A lack of community engagement and empowerment is a systemic barrier that undermines the success of interventions in food deserts. Marginalized populations often face barriers in participating in decision-making processes, limiting their ability to influence policies and programs that affect their access to healthy food.

To address this barrier, efforts must be made to empower and engage community members in decision-making processes. Community organizations and grassroots movements play a crucial role in promoting community participation and advocating for policy changes. Establishing community advisory boards, hosting public forums, and conducting outreach programs can help ensure that the voices of the marginalized are heard and their needs are addressed.

Racial and Social Inequalities

Racial and social inequalities are deeply intertwined with food deserts, perpetuating systemic barriers that limit access to healthy food. Communities of color and low-income communities are disproportionately affected by food deserts, reflecting broader social and economic disparities.

Addressing these inequalities requires approaches that tackle systemic racism and economic injustice. This includes advocating for policies that promote equitable distribution of resources, addressing discriminatory practices in the food industry, and promoting social and economic inclusion in food desert interventions. Additionally, educational programs and initiatives can raise awareness about the intersectionality of race, poverty, and food access, fostering a better understanding of the systemic barriers at play.

Conclusion

Systemic barriers form the foundation of food deserts and hinder efforts to address them effectively. By acknowledging and addressing these barriers, we can develop more comprehensive and sustainable solutions that promote food justice and improve access to healthy food in marginalized communities. It requires a multi-faceted approach that tackles issues of investment, infrastructure, affordability, community empowerment, and racial and social inequalities. Only by addressing these systemic barriers can we truly create positive and lasting change in the fight against food deserts.

Sustaining interventions in the long term

Sustaining interventions in the long term is crucial for addressing the issue of food deserts effectively. While short-term solutions may provide temporary relief, lasting change requires continuous efforts and a comprehensive approach. In this section, we will explore strategies for sustaining interventions in the long term, considering the economic, social, and environmental aspects of food deserts.

Economic sustainability

One of the key challenges in sustaining interventions is ensuring economic viability. Many food desert interventions rely on external funding or grants, which may not be sustainable in the long run. To address this, it is important to explore models that promote self-sufficiency and economic growth within the community.

Entrepreneurship and local businesses: Encouraging entrepreneurship and supporting local businesses can create economic opportunities within food deserts. Start-ups and social enterprises can play a significant role in providing access to healthy food options. For example, community-owned grocery stores and farmers' markets can generate revenue and create employment opportunities.

Social enterprises and cooperative models: Collaborative approaches like social enterprises and cooperative models can help ensure the sustainability of interventions. These models involve community participation and shared ownership, which fosters a sense of ownership and responsibility. For instance, a food cooperative can be established where community members contribute resources, time, and skills to ensure the availability of healthy food options.

Public-private partnerships: Collaborations between the public and private sectors can enhance the sustainability of interventions. Public-private partnerships can leverage the expertise and resources of both sectors to develop innovative solutions. For instance, a government agency can partner with a local grocery chain to establish a store in a food desert, ensuring sustainable food access through a mutually beneficial arrangement.

Social sustainability

Sustaining interventions in the long term also requires addressing social factors that influence food access and choices within food deserts. Social sustainability involves fostering community engagement, building trust, and ensuring equitable access to resources.

Community engagement and empowerment: Involving the community in the decision-making process and implementation of interventions is crucial for sustaining long-term efforts. Engaging community members as active participants empowers them to take ownership of the interventions and increases the likelihood of success. Community meetings, workshops, and focus groups can provide platforms for open dialogue and collective decision-making.

Education and awareness: Education plays a vital role in sustaining interventions. Promoting nutrition education and awareness campaigns can empower individuals to make informed food choices. By increasing knowledge about the importance of healthy eating, the community can sustain long-term behavior change. Collaborations with local schools, community centers, and healthcare providers can facilitate nutrition education programs.

Social support systems: Social support systems can help sustain interventions by providing assistance to vulnerable populations within food deserts. Establishing food banks, meal delivery services, and community kitchens can ensure access to nutritious food for individuals facing economic or physical barriers. Additionally, fostering social connections and support networks can reduce social isolation and improve overall well-being.

Environmental sustainability

Considering the environmental impact is crucial for the long-term sustainability of food desert interventions. Addressing environmental sustainability involves promoting environmentally friendly practices and minimizing the ecological footprint of interventions.

Promoting local and sustainable food systems: Supporting local food production and sustainable farming practices can contribute to environmental sustainability. Encouraging community gardens, urban farming, and supporting local farmers can reduce dependency on long-distance transportation and promote the use of organic farming techniques. This not only provides access to fresh, healthy produce but also reduces the carbon footprint associated with food transportation.

Waste management and recycling: Implementing waste management and recycling programs can minimize the environmental impact of food deserts interventions. For example, composting food waste from community gardens or implementing recycling initiatives at grocery stores can reduce waste sent to landfills. These initiatives can be integrated into food desert interventions, promoting sustainability and environmental consciousness.

Energy-efficient infrastructure: Designing energy-efficient infrastructure can contribute to the long-term sustainability of interventions. For instance, using solar panels or energy-efficient appliances at community-owned grocery stores can reduce energy consumption and promote renewable energy sources. Implementing sustainable practices in infrastructure development ensures a long-lasting positive impact on both the environment and the community.

In conclusion, sustaining interventions in the long term requires a multi-faceted approach that addresses economic, social, and environmental sustainability. By promoting entrepreneurship, community engagement, and socially responsible practices, interventions can create long-term positive change in food deserts. Additionally, incorporating environmental sustainability measures ensures that interventions have a minimal impact on the environment. Empowering communities, fostering collaboration, and prioritizing sustainable practices will contribute to the lasting success of interventions in combating food deserts.

Lessons learned from unsuccessful interventions

In researching and addressing food deserts, it is essential to examine both successful and unsuccessful interventions. While much can be learned from successful initiatives, it is equally important to understand and analyze the reasons behind failures. By identifying the shortcomings of unsuccessful interventions, researchers, policymakers, and advocates can avoid repeating mistakes and develop more effective strategies to combat food deserts. In this section, we will delve into the lessons learned from unsuccessful interventions and explore the factors that contributed to their lack of success.

One of the main lessons learned from unsuccessful interventions is the failure to prioritize community engagement and empowerment. Many interventions in the past have focused solely on providing access to healthy food without considering the specific needs and aspirations of the community. It is crucial for initiatives to involve community members from the inception to ensure that their voices and perspectives are heard. By actively involving the community, interventions can be tailored to meet their unique needs and cultural preferences, increasing the likelihood of success.

Another common factor contributing to the failure of interventions is the lack of sustainability. Many unsuccessful interventions relied heavily on external funding and support, which often dwindled over time. This led to a lack of resources and the inability to sustain the intervention in the long term. To overcome this challenge, interventions should focus on building local capacity and fostering self-sufficiency within the community. By empowering community members to take ownership of the intervention and develop their skills, they can continue to address food deserts even after external support diminishes.

In some cases, unsuccessful interventions failed to address the root causes of food deserts, instead focusing solely on the symptoms. Without addressing the underlying issues such as poverty, income inequality, and systemic discrimination, interventions can only provide temporary relief. To achieve sustainable change, interventions must tackle the structural barriers that perpetuate food deserts. This could involve advocating for policy changes, promoting economic opportunities, and addressing social inequalities that contribute to food insecurity.

Another important lesson learned is the failure to consider the impact of cultural preferences and social dynamics within the community. Interventions that did not take into account the cultural and social norms of the community often faced resistance and lack of acceptance. To be successful, interventions should not only provide access to healthy food but also ensure that the food is culturally appropriate and aligns with the community's dietary preferences. Understanding the community's food traditions and incorporating them into interventions can help overcome barriers and enhance the likelihood of success.

Furthermore, unsuccessful interventions often overlooked the importance of comprehensive evaluation and continuous monitoring. Without robust evaluation methods, it is challenging to measure the effectiveness and impact of an intervention accurately. In some cases, interventions may have appeared successful initially but failed to maintain the desired outcomes in the long term. By implementing rigorous evaluation strategies, interventions can identify early warning signs and make necessary adjustments to improve effectiveness.

An important lesson learned from unsuccessful interventions is the need for collaboration and coordination among various stakeholders. Lack of collaboration can lead to duplication of efforts, inefficient use of resources, and fragmented interventions. Collaborative efforts involving government agencies, non-profit organizations, local businesses, community members, and researchers can leverage collective expertise and resources to develop holistic and sustainable solutions. By fostering partnerships and creating interdisciplinary networks, interventions can maximize their impact and achieve long-term success.

In conclusion, analyzing the failures of past interventions is crucial for understanding and addressing food deserts effectively. By examining the lessons learned from unsuccessful interventions, we can avoid repeating mistakes and develop more sustainable, culturally appropriate, and community-driven strategies. Prioritizing community engagement, sustainability, addressing root causes, considering cultural preferences, implementing comprehensive evaluations, and fostering collaboration are key factors in successful interventions that aim to eliminate food deserts and promote food justice.

Equity and Social Justice in Interventions

Ensuring equitable access to healthy food

In addressing the issue of food deserts, it is crucial to prioritize equitable access to healthy food for all individuals. This section explores various strategies and approaches to ensure that everyone has the opportunity to obtain nutritious food regardless of their socioeconomic status, race, or location.

The Importance of Equitable Access

Equitable access to healthy food is a fundamental aspect of achieving food justice. It recognizes the rights of individuals to have equal opportunities for food security and nutrition. When access to nutritious food is unequal, it exacerbates existing social inequalities and perpetuates health disparities.

A key principle in ensuring equitable access is the recognition that everyone should have physical and financial access to a variety of healthy foods that meet their dietary needs. This includes affordable fresh fruits and vegetables, whole grains, lean proteins, and dairy products. Achieving equitable access involves addressing the multiple barriers that different populations face in accessing healthy food options.

Addressing Barriers to Equitable Access

To ensure equitable access to healthy food, it is essential to identify and address the barriers that prevent certain populations from obtaining nutritious food. These barriers may include:

- **Physical barriers:** Limited availability of grocery stores or farmers markets in low-income neighborhoods, lack of transportation options, and long distances to the nearest food retailer.

- **Financial barriers:** High cost of nutritious foods compared to high-calorie, low-nutrient options, limited food budgets, and lack of affordable grocery options in food deserts.

- **Social and cultural barriers:** Limited awareness and education about nutrition, lack of cooking skills, and cultural preferences for unhealthy foods. Language barriers can also impact access for non-English speaking communities.

- **Policy and structural barriers:** Zoning regulations that limit the establishment of grocery stores in certain areas, inadequate infrastructure for food distribution, and discriminatory practices in food retail.

To address these barriers and promote equitable access, a comprehensive approach is needed, involving stakeholders from government, community organizations, and the private sector.

Policy Solutions

Policy changes and interventions play a crucial role in ensuring equitable access to healthy food. Some key strategies include:

- **Improving food retail in underserved areas:** Local governments can offer incentives for grocery stores to open in food deserts or provide additional support for existing retailers in these areas. This can include tax incentives, grants, or loans to help overcome the financial challenges of operating in underserved communities.

- **Mobile markets and food delivery services:** Mobile markets and food delivery services can bridge the gap in areas where access to grocery stores is limited. These initiatives can bring fresh produce and other healthy food options directly to communities in need.

- **Healthy food financing initiatives:** Governments can establish loan programs or grants to support the development of grocery stores, food co-ops, or farmers markets in underserved areas. This can help address the financial barriers associated with opening and operating food retail establishments in low-income neighborhoods.

Community-Based Approaches

Community-based approaches are instrumental in addressing food access inequities. These approaches empower local communities to take ownership of their food systems and prioritize the needs of their residents. Examples of community-based approaches include:

- **Community gardens and urban farming:** Community gardens and urban farming initiatives allow individuals to grow their own food, increasing access to fresh produce. These initiatives also provide opportunities for education and community building.

- **Farmers markets and food cooperatives:** Farmers markets and food cooperatives create direct connections between local farmers and consumers. They promote sustainable food systems and offer affordable, fresh, and culturally appropriate food options.

- **Community food assessments:** Conducting community food assessments can help identify specific areas within a community where access to healthy food is lacking. This information can inform targeted interventions and initiatives.

Education and Empowerment

Education and empowerment initiatives are essential components of promoting equitable access to healthy food. These initiatives aim to increase awareness, knowledge, and skills related to nutrition, cooking, and food choices.

- **Nutrition education in schools and communities:** Integrating nutrition education into school curricula and community programs can empower individuals to make informed food choices. This includes teaching essential skills like meal planning, budgeting, and cooking.

- **Public health campaigns:** Public health campaigns raise awareness about the importance of healthy eating and the impact of food deserts on community health. These campaigns can target specific populations and work to change perceptions and behaviors.

- **Promoting local food systems:** Educating communities about the benefits of supporting local food systems can foster a sense of community pride and emphasize the importance of sustainable food production and consumption.

Advocacy and Collaboration

Advocacy and collaboration are critical in driving systemic change and ensuring long-term equitable access to healthy food. Key strategies in this regard include:

- **Building partnerships and collaborations:** Collaborations between governments, community organizations, non-profits, and private entities can leverage resources, expertise, and influence to address food access inequalities. These partnerships help foster sustainable solutions and amplify the impact of interventions.

- **Policy advocacy:** Advocacy efforts can play a significant role in promoting policy changes that address the root causes of food deserts. This includes advocating for legislation that supports equitable access, funding for interventions, and changes to zoning regulations.

- **Social mobilization:** Grassroots movements and community organizing can amplify the voices of communities affected by food deserts. By mobilizing individuals and collectively advocating for change, communities can create lasting impact and hold decision-makers accountable.

Conclusion

Ensuring equitable access to healthy food is a multifaceted challenge that requires a holistic and collaborative approach. By addressing the barriers to access, implementing policy changes, empowering communities, and advocating for systemic change, we can work towards achieving food justice. It is essential to prioritize equity in all interventions, policies, and programs to create a more just and inclusive food system.

Social and Economic Inclusion in Interventions

Social and economic inclusion are crucial elements when designing interventions to address food deserts. These interventions aim to improve access to healthy and affordable food options for all individuals, regardless of their socio-economic status or background. In this section, we will explore the importance of social and economic inclusion in interventions, discuss strategies for promoting inclusivity, and highlight the benefits of ensuring equitable access to healthy food.

Importance of Social and Economic Inclusion

In the context of food deserts, social and economic inclusion refers to creating interventions that cater to the diverse needs of the community, including individuals with limited financial resources, minority populations, and marginalized groups. It recognizes that food access and affordability are deeply intertwined with social and economic factors.

Social inclusion involves ensuring that all individuals, irrespective of their social identities, have equal opportunities and resources to obtain healthy food. Economic inclusion, on the other hand, focuses on addressing the financial barriers that prevent individuals from accessing nutritious food. By prioritizing social and economic inclusion, interventions can effectively target the root causes of food deserts and improve overall health and well-being.

Strategies for Promoting Inclusivity

To promote social and economic inclusion in interventions addressing food deserts, various strategies can be employed:

1. Community Engagement: Engaging with the community is essential to understand their specific needs and challenges. This can be achieved through active participation, listening sessions, surveys, and focus groups. It allows community members to contribute their thoughts and ideas, ensuring that interventions are culturally relevant and meet the needs of the diverse population.

2. Collaborative Partnerships: Building collaborations with local organizations, community groups, and stakeholders is crucial for inclusivity. These partnerships can help mobilize resources, increase community participation, and ensure that interventions are tailored to meet the unique needs of the community.

3. Targeted Funding and Resources: Allocating targeted funding and resources to areas with high food desert prevalence and low-income communities is essential. This ensures that interventions are accessible to those who need them the most and can help alleviate the financial burden of accessing healthy food.

4. Culturally Tailored Interventions: Understanding and respecting cultural norms, dietary preferences, and food traditions is important in designing effective interventions. By incorporating culturally appropriate strategies, such as offering diverse food options and promoting traditional recipes, interventions can better engage and meet the needs of the community.

5. Addressing Language and Literacy Barriers: Interventions should consider language and literacy barriers by providing information and resources in multiple languages and formats. This ensures that individuals with limited English proficiency or low literacy levels can access and understand the information provided.

Benefits of Social and Economic Inclusion

Promoting social and economic inclusion in interventions has several benefits:

1. Health Equity: Social and economic inclusion helps bridge the health disparities related to food access. By ensuring that all individuals have access to healthy food options, interventions can promote health equity and reduce the risk of diet-related diseases.

2. Community Ownership and Empowerment: Inclusive interventions empower the community by involving them in the decision-making process. This sense of ownership increases the likelihood of sustainable solutions and fosters community pride and cohesion.

3. Economic Development: Inclusive interventions can stimulate local economic growth by supporting local farmers, food producers, and entrepreneurs. By creating opportunities for collaboration and entrepreneurship, interventions can contribute to a vibrant local food economy and job creation.

4. Social Cohesion: Inclusive interventions promote social cohesion by fostering constructive relationships across different socio-economic and cultural backgrounds. This enhances community resilience and social capital, leading to a stronger and more connected community.

In conclusion, social and economic inclusion are integral to designing effective interventions to address food deserts. By prioritizing inclusivity, interventions can better understand and address the unique needs of diverse communities. Strategies such as community engagement, collaborative partnerships, targeted funding, and culturally tailored interventions can promote social and economic inclusion, leading to better health outcomes and a more equitable food system.

Advocating for Systemic Change and Social Justice

Advocating for systemic change and social justice is a crucial component of addressing food deserts. While individual interventions can make a difference, they often fail to tackle the root causes of food inequality. In this section, we will explore the importance of advocacy in creating lasting change, strategies for advocating for systemic change, and the role of social justice in achieving food justice.

Understanding Systemic Change

Systemic change refers to large-scale transformations that aim to challenge and alter the underlying structures and systems that perpetuate inequality. In the context of food deserts, systemic change involves challenging economic, social, and political factors that contribute to the creation and persistence of food deserts.

To effectively advocate for systemic change, it is important to understand the interconnectedness of various factors that contribute to food deserts. This includes recognizing the influence of economic disparities, racial and ethnic inequalities, urban planning policies, and the food industry's practices. Systemic change requires addressing these factors holistically and creating an environment that supports equitable access to healthy food for all.

Strategies for Advocating for Systemic Change

Advocacy for systemic change can take many forms and requires collaboration among various stakeholders. Here are some strategies that can be employed to advocate for systemic change in relation to food deserts:

1. Policy advocacy: Engage with policymakers at local, state, and national levels to develop and implement policies that address food deserts. This may involve advocating for zoning regulations that support grocery store development

in underserved areas or securing funding for community-based programs that promote food access.

2. Public awareness campaigns: Raise public awareness about the issue of food deserts and the importance of equitable access to healthy food. Use various platforms such as social media, community events, and educational campaigns to disseminate information and mobilize support for systemic change.

3. Coalition building: Collaborate with other organizations, community groups, and individuals working towards social justice to amplify voices and share resources. By forming coalitions, advocates can join forces to advocate for policy changes and influence decision-makers.

4. Engage the food industry: Encourage food retailers, distributors, and manufacturers to address food deserts by investing in underserved areas and providing healthier food options. Advocate for partnerships between the public and private sectors to create sustainable solutions.

5. Grassroots organizing: Empower communities affected by food deserts to advocate for their own needs. Support community-led initiatives, such as community gardens and food cooperatives, that empower residents to take control of their food environment and demand systemic change.

The Role of Social Justice in Achieving Food Justice

Social justice is a fundamental principle in advocating for food justice. Addressing food deserts requires acknowledging and addressing the underlying social and economic inequalities that create and perpetuate food disparities. By adopting a social justice framework, advocates seek to ensure equitable access to healthy food for all individuals, regardless of their socio-economic status, race, or ethnicity.

Social justice requires dismantling the systemic barriers that contribute to food inequality. This includes challenging policies and practices that perpetuate food deserts, advocating for fair wages and employment opportunities, addressing racial and ethnic disparities in food access, and promoting inclusive community development.

In advocating for social justice, it is crucial to prioritize the voices of marginalized communities and involve them in decision-making processes. This includes centering the experiences and knowledge of those directly affected by food deserts and incorporating their perspectives into policy development and implementation.

Achieving social justice in the context of food deserts requires a collective effort that extends beyond individual actions. By advocating for systemic change and embracing social justice principles, we can work towards a future where everyone has equal access to nutritious food, regardless of where they live or their socio-economic standing.

Real-World Example: The Healthy Chicago Initiative

The Healthy Chicago Initiative is an example of advocacy for systemic change and social justice in addressing food deserts. Initiated by the City of Chicago in response to the prevalence of food deserts in certain neighborhoods, the initiative aims to improve access to healthy food and promote community development.

The initiative adopts a multi-pronged approach, involving collaboration between government agencies, community organizations, and residents. It focuses on implementing policies that support the development of grocery stores in underserved areas, providing financial incentives to retailers, and improving transportation infrastructure to enhance food access.

Additionally, the Healthy Chicago Initiative actively engages with community members through public forums, surveys, and community-led initiatives. This ensures that the voices and perspectives of the affected communities are directly incorporated into decision-making processes.

The initiative also recognizes the importance of social justice in achieving food justice. It aims to address the underlying social and economic factors that contribute to food deserts, including income disparities, racial inequalities, and limited employment opportunities.

By advocating for systemic change and embracing social justice principles, the Healthy Chicago Initiative serves as a model for addressing food deserts in a comprehensive and equitable manner.

Summary

Advocating for systemic change and social justice is vital for addressing food deserts effectively. By understanding the interconnectedness of various factors contributing to food inequality, employing strategies for systemic change, and embracing social justice principles, we can work towards creating a future where everyone has equal access to healthy and nutritious food. Through concerted efforts, collaboration, and inclusive decision-making processes, we can advocate for lasting change and achieve food justice for all.

Future Trends and Directions in Food Desert Research

Emerging Topics and Areas of Interest

Climate Change and Food Deserts

Climate change is a global crisis that is significantly impacting various aspects of our lives, including access to nutritious food. The interplay between climate change and food deserts presents significant challenges for addressing food insecurity and ensuring equitable access to healthy food options. In this section, we will explore the relationship between climate change and food deserts, examine the implications for vulnerable populations, and discuss potential strategies to mitigate the impact.

Rising Temperatures and Crop Production

One of the primary effects of climate change is rising temperatures, which pose a threat to crop production. Higher temperatures can result in reduced yields and productivity for staple crops such as wheat, rice, and maize. This can exacerbate the existing challenges faced by communities living in food deserts, where access to fresh produce is already limited.

For example, in regions with already limited agricultural resources, such as arid and semi-arid areas, increases in temperature can lead to drought conditions and desertification. This not only reduces the availability of locally grown food but also increases the reliance on food transportation, leading to an increase in carbon emissions and exacerbating the climate crisis further.

Extreme Weather Events and Supply Chain Disruptions

Climate change is also associated with an increase in the frequency and intensity of extreme weather events, such as hurricanes, floods, and droughts. These events can disrupt the entire food supply chain, from production to distribution, and exacerbate food insecurity in already vulnerable communities.

In food deserts, where access to nutritious food is already limited, extreme weather events can have devastating consequences. For instance, a flood can destroy crops, making it even more difficult for local communities to access fresh produce. Similarly, hurricanes can damage transportation infrastructure, making it challenging to transport food from outside the area.

Sea-Level Rise and Coastal Food Deserts

Sea-level rise, another consequence of climate change, poses a significant threat to coastal regions and can contribute to the emergence of coastal food deserts. As sea levels rise, fertile agricultural lands near the coast become saline and unsuitable for farming. This loss of arable land further limits the availability of locally sourced fresh produce, forcing coastal communities to rely on imported food.

Coastal food deserts also face the risk of contamination of freshwater sources, leading to reduced availability of clean water for irrigation and consumption. Disruptions in the local fishing industry due to changes in ocean currents and loss of marine biodiversity further compound the challenges faced by these communities.

Mitigating the Impact

Addressing the intersection of climate change and food deserts requires a multi-faceted approach that combines strategies for climate mitigation and adaptation with initiatives to improve food access and community resilience. Here are some potential strategies that can help mitigate the impact:

1. Sustainable Agriculture Practices Promoting sustainable agriculture practices, such as agroecology and organic farming, can help reduce greenhouse gas emissions, conserve water resources, and improve soil health. These practices can enhance the resilience of food systems to climate change and increase the availability of locally grown, nutritious food in food deserts.

2. Climate-Resilient Infrastructure Investing in climate-resilient infrastructure, such as flood-resistant storage facilities and transportation networks, can help minimize disruptions in the food supply chain during extreme weather events. This infrastructure should be designed to withstand climate-related risks and ensure the continued availability of fresh and healthy food in food deserts.

3. Diversifying Food Sources Diversifying food sources through the promotion of alternative crops and food production methods can protect against crop failures caused by climate change. For instance, incorporating climate-resilient crops that are better adapted to changing weather patterns can help ensure a stable food supply in regions susceptible to extreme weather events.

4. Enhancing Food Storage and Preservation Improving food storage and preservation techniques can help reduce food waste and ensure a more reliable food supply in food deserts. This includes implementing efficient cold storage facilities and promoting community-led initiatives such as canning, drying, and fermenting foods to extend their shelf life.

5. Community Resilience and Education Building community resilience and providing education on climate change and food systems is essential for addressing the climate-food desert nexus. This includes empowering community members with knowledge and skills to adapt to changing environmental conditions, fostering local food production initiatives, and advocating for policy changes that prioritize food justice and climate action.

Case Study: The Gambia

In the West African country of The Gambia, climate change poses significant challenges to food security, particularly in rural areas. Rising temperatures and erratic rainfall patterns have led to unpredictable growing seasons and reduced crop yields, exacerbating food insecurity in communities already facing limited access to fresh and nutritious food.

To address this issue, the government of The Gambia, in collaboration with international organizations and local communities, has implemented various strategies. These include promoting climate-smart agriculture techniques, such as agroforestry and conservation farming, to enhance agricultural productivity and resilience to climate change. The government has also invested in rural infrastructure development, including improved irrigation systems and roads, to facilitate the transportation of food to remote areas.

Furthermore, community-led initiatives, such as women's farming cooperatives and community gardens, have been established to empower local communities and improve access to fresh produce. These initiatives not only promote sustainable food production but also enhance community resilience by providing alternative sources of income and nutrition.

The case of The Gambia highlights the importance of implementing integrated approaches that combine climate mitigation and adaptation strategies with community engagement and empowerment. By addressing the challenges posed by climate change and food deserts holistically, it is possible to build more resilient and equitable food systems.

Conclusion

The interaction between climate change and food deserts presents significant challenges for ensuring food security and equity. Rising temperatures, extreme weather events, and sea-level rise all contribute to the vulnerability of marginalized communities living in food deserts. However, through sustainable agriculture practices, climate-resilient infrastructure, diversification of food sources, food storage and preservation techniques, and community resilience and education, it is possible to mitigate the impact of climate change on food deserts.

By taking a comprehensive and interdisciplinary approach, involving governments, communities, and international organizations, we can work towards building resilient and equitable food systems that are capable of withstanding the challenges posed by climate change. It is essential to prioritize the needs of those most affected by climate change, ensuring that the solutions we develop are inclusive, sustainable, and just. Let us commit to addressing climate change and food deserts hand in hand and create a future where everyone has access to healthy and nutritious food, regardless of their geographical location.

Effects of COVID-19 on food access

The COVID-19 pandemic has had a profound impact on various aspects of our lives, including the food system. The global health crisis has disrupted supply chains, limited access to resources, and exacerbated existing inequalities in food access. In this section, we will explore the effects of COVID-19 on food access, examining both the immediate challenges faced during the pandemic and the long-term implications for addressing food deserts.

Immediate Challenges

When the pandemic hit, it led to widespread closures of businesses and institutions, including restaurants, schools, and food markets. These closures disrupted the traditional avenues through which people obtained their food, leaving many individuals without easy access to fresh and nutritious options.

One immediate challenge was the sudden increase in food insecurity. As millions of people lost their jobs or experienced reduced income, they were unable to afford an adequate diet. This resulted in a surge in demand for food banks and other emergency food assistance programs. However, many of these organizations faced shortages of resources and struggled to meet the heightened need.

Additionally, the pandemic highlighted the limitations of relying on traditional brick-and-mortar grocery stores, especially for vulnerable populations in food deserts. With stay-at-home orders and concerns about public gatherings, people were hesitant to visit crowded supermarkets. For those who lacked reliable transportation or lived in areas with limited grocery options, the closure of stores exacerbated existing challenges in accessing nutritious food.

Supply Chain Disruptions

A significant contributing factor to the challenges faced during the pandemic was the disruption of the food supply chain. Lockdown measures, travel restrictions, and labor shortages affected the production, processing, and distribution of food. Farmers faced difficulties in harvesting crops due to a lack of available workers, as well as disruption in the transportation of goods to markets.

The closure of restaurants and hotels, which traditionally accounted for a significant portion of food demand, led to a surplus of products, particularly perishable items such as fruits and vegetables. Simultaneously, panic buying and stockpiling by consumers resulted in shortages of staple items like rice, pasta, and canned goods.

These disruptions in the supply chain highlighted vulnerabilities and inefficiencies in our food system, further exacerbating unequal access to fresh and affordable food.

Long-term Implications

While the immediate challenges posed by COVID-19 were significant, the long-term implications are equally concerning. The pandemic exposed the vulnerabilities and inequalities within our food system, particularly in food deserts.

Firstly, the economic fallout from the pandemic will likely have lasting effects on food access. As unemployment rates rise and economic disparities widen, affordability becomes a critical issue. Many individuals, especially those already living in poverty or low-income households, may struggle to meet their basic food needs.

Secondly, the closure of local businesses, including grocery stores, during the pandemic may have long-lasting consequences for food access in underserved areas. Without intervention, these closures could result in a further concentration of food deserts, making it even more challenging for residents to access healthier options.

Thirdly, the shift towards online food purchasing and delivery services during the pandemic creates a new set of challenges. While these services offer convenience and flexibility, they can also perpetuate disparities in food access. Many low-income individuals may lack reliable internet access or credit cards required for online purchases, further marginalizing them from the benefits of these services.

Addressing the Challenges

To address the effects of COVID-19 on food access, it is crucial to adopt a multi-faceted approach that combines immediate measures and long-term strategies. Here are some potential solutions and interventions:

- Strengthening emergency food assistance programs: Ensuring that food banks and other emergency food providers have sufficient resources to meet the increased demand is critical. This includes financial support, logistics assistance, and coordination with local community organizations.

- Investing in local and regional food systems: Supporting local farmers, farmers markets, and community-supported agriculture (CSA) programs can help diversify the food supply chain and reduce dependence on large-scale distribution networks. This not only improves food access but also enhances the resilience of the local economy.

- Expanding transportation options: Addressing transportation barriers in food deserts is crucial for improving access to nutritious food. This includes investing in public transportation infrastructure, promoting ridesharing initiatives, and establishing mobile markets or food delivery services in underserved areas.

- Increasing affordability and access to healthy food: Implementing policies to lower the cost of nutritious food, such as subsidies or incentives for purchasing fruits and vegetables, can help alleviate economic barriers. Additionally, expanding the availability of affordable fresh produce through initiatives like urban farming or community gardens can have a significant impact.

- Enhancing digital inclusion: To mitigate the inequities in online food purchasing, efforts should be made to improve digital literacy and accessibility, bridging the digital divide. This can involve providing internet access in underserved communities and educational programs on using online platforms effectively.

By implementing these interventions, we can begin to address the immediate challenges faced during the pandemic and work towards long-term solutions for improving food access in the face of future crises.

Conclusion

The COVID-19 pandemic has highlighted and exacerbated the inequalities within our food system, particularly in food deserts. The immediate challenges of food insecurity, supply chain disruptions, and limitations in food access have long-lasting implications for vulnerable populations.

Addressing the effects of COVID-19 on food access requires a comprehensive approach that combines emergency measures with long-term strategies. By investing in local food systems, improving transportation options, enhancing affordability, and promoting digital inclusion, we can begin to build a more resilient and equitable food system.

Moving forward, it is crucial to learn from the lessons of the pandemic and work towards systemic changes that address the root causes of food deserts. By doing so, we can build a future where everyone has access to affordable, nutritious, and culturally appropriate food, regardless of their socioeconomic status or geographic location.

Innovative solutions for the future

As we look toward the future, addressing the issue of food deserts requires innovative solutions that combine technological advancements, community engagement, and policy changes. In this section, we will explore some of the exciting and promising approaches that hold potential for improving food access and nutrition in underserved communities.

Mobile applications for food access

Mobile applications have become an integral part of our daily lives, providing convenience and accessibility to a wide range of services. In the context of food deserts, mobile applications can play a crucial role in connecting residents with healthy food options. These apps can provide various features, including:

- **Store locator:** GPS-enabled maps that help users find the nearest grocery stores, farmers markets, or community gardens.
- **Product information:** Providing detailed information about the nutritional value, ingredients, and sourcing of food products to facilitate informed choices.
- **Price comparisons:** Allowing users to compare prices of essential food items across different stores to make budget-friendly decisions.
- **Inventory updates:** Real-time updates on food availability and promotions to ensure that users have accurate information before making a trip to the store.
- **Community networks:** Creating platforms for users to share their experiences, recommendations, and potential solutions for addressing food deserts in their community.

By harnessing the accessibility of smartphones, these applications have the potential to empower individuals to make healthier food choices and navigate their local food landscape more effectively.

Online platforms for food delivery

In recent years, online grocery shopping and food delivery services have gained significant popularity. These platforms offer convenience, especially for individuals with limited mobility or transportation options. To address food deserts, online platforms can be specifically tailored to prioritize underserved communities and provide affordable, healthy food options. Some potential features of such platforms include:

- **Localized delivery services:** Collaborating with local grocery stores, farmers, and distributors to ensure timely and affordable deliveries to food desert areas.
- **Subsidized pricing:** Offering discounted prices or subsidies on fresh produce and staple food items for individuals living in food deserts.

- **Nutrition guidance:** Providing personalized nutrition recommendations and meal planning assistance to promote healthier choices among users.
- **Community engagement:** Facilitating virtual interaction and engagement through online forums, webinars, and social media platforms to create a sense of community and support.
- **Data-driven solutions:** Utilizing data analytics to identify patterns of food preferences and demands, and tailoring offerings accordingly to address the specific needs of each food desert community.

By leveraging the power of e-commerce, these platforms can revolutionize the way food is accessed and distributed in underserved areas.

Vertical farming and urban agriculture

With limited space and resources in urban environments, traditional agriculture may be challenging in food desert areas. However, innovative farming methods, such as vertical farming and urban agriculture, offer promising solutions. These approaches allow for the cultivation of crops in controlled indoor environments, using advanced technologies like hydroponics or aeroponics. Benefits of these techniques include:

- **Year-round production:** Vertical farming systems can provide a consistent supply of fresh produce throughout the year, reducing dependence on seasonal availability.
- **Spatial efficiency:** By utilizing vertical space, these systems can maximize productivity in urban areas with limited land availability.
- **Reduced environmental impact:** Vertical farming requires less water and land compared to traditional agriculture, making it a sustainable option for food production.
- **Community involvement:** Engaging local residents in urban farming initiatives can foster a sense of community and improve food literacy.
- **Educational opportunities:** Integrating urban agriculture into school curricula can provide hands-on learning experiences and promote healthy eating habits among children.

While vertical farming and urban agriculture are still evolving practices, they hold immense potential for increasing food production and accessibility in densely populated food desert areas.

Blockchain technology for transparent food systems

Transparency and traceability are essential in ensuring the quality and safety of food products. Blockchain technology, which offers a decentralized and immutable record of transactions, can be leveraged to create transparent food systems. By using blockchain, we can:

- **Enhance food safety:** Blockchain can track the entire supply chain, reducing the risk of contamination and fraudulent practices.
- **Ensure fair trade:** Smart contracts on blockchain can create fair payment systems and provide better visibility into the distribution of profits among farmers, suppliers, and retailers.
- **Promote sustainable practices:** Blockchain can enable the certification and verification of eco-friendly farming techniques and fair labor practices, encouraging more sustainable food production.
- **Empower consumer choice:** With transparent information about the origin and production methods of food products, consumers can make more informed and conscious choices.

By ensuring transparency and trust, blockchain technology can promote healthier and more equitable food systems, benefiting both producers and consumers in food desert communities.

Engaging the private sector

Collaboration with the private sector is crucial in developing sustainable and scalable solutions for food deserts. By involving large food retailers, tech companies, and investors, innovative approaches can gain the necessary resources and expertise. Some potential avenues for private sector involvement include:

- **Public-private partnerships:** Collaborating with private entities to establish affordable grocery stores, farmers markets, or mobile food trucks in underserved areas.
- **Corporate social responsibility:** Encouraging corporations to allocate resources and investments toward addressing food deserts as part of their social responsibility initiatives.

- **Tech innovation support:** Partnering with technology and innovation companies to develop and implement advanced solutions like mobile apps, online platforms, or data analytics for food desert communities.
- **Social impact investing:** Mobilizing private capital to fund sustainable and impactful projects that target food desert areas, including urban agriculture ventures or community-owned grocery stores.

By fostering collaboration between the public and private sectors, innovative solutions can be effectively implemented and scaled, leading to long-term positive outcomes for food desert communities.

Conclusion

Innovative solutions hold tremendous potential for addressing the complex issue of food deserts. Through mobile applications, online platforms, vertical farming, blockchain technology, and collaborations with the private sector, we can create lasting changes in food access and nutrition in underserved communities. However, it is crucial to approach these solutions with a holistic, community-centered perspective, considering the unique challenges and opportunities each food desert presents. By combining innovation, interdisciplinary collaboration, and a commitment to equity and social justice, we can work towards a future where equal access to healthy food is a reality for all.

Interdisciplinary Approaches to Food Desert Research

Collaborative Research Across Disciplines

Collaborative research across disciplines is a crucial approach to tackling complex issues such as food deserts. It involves bringing together experts from different fields to combine their knowledge, skills, and perspectives in order to generate innovative and comprehensive solutions. In this section, we will explore the benefits of interdisciplinary collaboration, the challenges it presents, and strategies for successful integration.

Benefits of Interdisciplinary Collaboration

Interdisciplinary collaboration offers numerous benefits in addressing the complex problems associated with food deserts. By fusing expertise from various disciplines, researchers can gain a more holistic understanding of the underlying factors contributing to food deserts and develop comprehensive solutions. Some key benefits include:

1. **Diverse Perspectives:** Different disciplines approach problems from unique angles, bringing diverse perspectives that can enrich the research process. For example, nutritionists can provide insights into the nutritional impact of food deserts, while urban planners can offer expertise on spatial distribution and transportation access.

2. **Creative Problem Solving:** Interdisciplinary teams often foster creativity and innovation by encouraging individuals to think outside their traditional disciplinary boundaries. This can lead to novel approaches and interventions that may not have been considered within a single discipline.

3. **Synergistic Collaboration:** Collaborating across disciplines allows researchers to leverage complementary skills and knowledge. This synergy can lead to more effective research outcomes and a deeper understanding of the complexities of food deserts.

4. **Comprehensive Solutions:** Food deserts require comprehensive solutions that address multiple factors simultaneously. Interdisciplinary research can facilitate the integration of findings from different fields, leading to more holistic interventions that tackle various dimensions of the problem.

Challenges of Interdisciplinary Collaboration

While interdisciplinary collaboration brings significant benefits, it also presents challenges that must be addressed to ensure effective teamwork and research outcomes. Some common challenges include:

1. **Communication Barriers:** Each discipline has its own jargon, methodologies, and ways of thinking. Effective communication can be hindered when researchers from different disciplines struggle to understand and articulate ideas clearly. Overcoming these barriers requires patience, active listening, and the use of shared language.

2. **Power Dynamics:** Collaborations may involve researchers from different levels of seniority and authority within their respective disciplines. Balancing power dynamics and creating an inclusive environment where all members' voices are heard is essential for productive interdisciplinary collaboration.

3. **Time and Resource Constraints:** Interdisciplinary research often requires additional time and resources compared to single-discipline research. Coordinating schedules, securing funding, and managing interdisciplinary teams can be resource-intensive. However, these challenges can be mitigated through careful planning, effective project management, and leveraging existing infrastructures.

4. **Methodological Differences:** Different disciplines often employ different research methods, which may lead to conflicts or difficulty in harmonizing methodologies. Finding common ground and adopting complementary approaches can help overcome these challenges.

Strategies for Successful Integration

To foster successful interdisciplinary collaboration in food desert research, certain strategies can be employed. These strategies include:

1. **Establishing a Common Goal:** Clearly defining a shared goal or research question provides a unifying focus for the interdisciplinary team. This common purpose helps align efforts and encourages collaboration.

2. **Building Interdisciplinary Teams:** Assembling interdisciplinary teams with individuals from diverse backgrounds and areas of expertise is essential. Each team member should bring unique perspectives, skills, and knowledge to contribute to the research project.

3. **Promoting Effective Communication:** Open and effective communication is critical for interdisciplinary collaboration. Creating spaces for regular dialogue, such as team meetings or virtual platforms, can help foster shared understanding and trust among team members.

4. **Facilitating Cross-Disciplinary Training:** Providing opportunities for team members to learn about each other's disciplines can enhance collaboration. Workshops, seminars, or training sessions can facilitate knowledge exchange and help researchers develop a common understanding of different disciplinary approaches.

5. **Integrating Multiple Disciplines' Methods:** Combining methodologies from different disciplines offers a more comprehensive approach to food desert research. By integrating data collection, analysis techniques, and theoretical frameworks, researchers can gain a deeper understanding of food deserts and their implications.

6. **Emphasizing Mutual Respect and Inclusion:** Valuing and respecting the expertise of all team members creates an inclusive environment for interdisciplinary collaboration. Encouraging active participation and recognizing each discipline's unique contributions fosters a culture of respect and appreciation.

Case Study: Interdisciplinary Research on Food Access and Urban Planning

To illustrate the power of interdisciplinary collaboration, let's consider a case study that combines the fields of food access and urban planning. In this study, researchers from nutrition, public health, transportation, and urban planning disciplines collaborated to understand the relationship between food access and urban design in an underserved neighborhood.

The team initially conducted a survey to assess the food access landscape and identify barriers faced by residents. The nutrition and public health experts analyzed the survey data to determine the nutritional implications of limited food access, while the transportation and urban planning experts examined the neighborhood's infrastructure and transportation systems.

Through interdisciplinary discussions, the team discovered that poor transportation connectivity was a significant barrier to accessing healthy food options. They proposed several solutions, including improving public transportation routes and creating bicycle lanes to connect the neighborhood to nearby grocery stores. Additionally, the urban planning experts suggested redesigning public spaces to incorporate community gardens and farmers markets.

By integrating their findings and expertise, the interdisciplinary team developed a comprehensive intervention plan that addressed both the nutritional and infrastructural dimensions of food deserts. Their collaborative efforts resulted in actionable recommendations that could be implemented by local policymakers and community organizations to improve food access and health outcomes in the underserved neighborhood.

Resources for Interdisciplinary Research

Engaging in interdisciplinary research requires access to relevant resources and knowledge from various disciplines. Some useful resources for researchers interested in interdisciplinary work on food deserts include:

- **Interdisciplinary Journals:** Journals such as *Interdisciplinary Food Studies* and *Journal of Urban Health* publish research at the intersection of multiple disciplines, providing a platform for interdisciplinary scholars to share their work.

- **Interdisciplinary Conferences and Workshops:** Attending interdisciplinary conferences and workshops, such as the International Symposium on Food Security and Nutrition or the Urban Affairs Association Annual Conference, offers opportunities to connect with researchers from different fields, learn about interdisciplinary work, and present research findings.
- **Interdisciplinary Research Centers and Institutes:** Many universities have research centers or institutes dedicated to interdisciplinary work. These centers often provide resources, funding opportunities, and networking platforms for interdisciplinary researchers.
- **Collaborative Grant Programs:** Funding agencies increasingly prioritize interdisciplinary research. Collaborative grant programs, such as the National Science Foundation's Integrative Strategies for Understanding Neural and Cognitive Systems program, can provide financial support for interdisciplinary research projects.

Remember, successful interdisciplinary collaboration requires openness, flexibility, and a willingness to learn from others. By embracing the challenges and benefits of interdisciplinary research, we can advance our understanding of food deserts and develop effective strategies to address this critical issue.

Exercises

1. Identify two disciplines outside of nutrition and public health that could contribute to interdisciplinary research on food deserts. Explain how each discipline's expertise could inform our understanding of food deserts and potential solutions.

2. Imagine you are part of an interdisciplinary team studying food deserts. How would you approach resolving communication barriers between team members from different disciplines? Provide at least three strategies to promote effective communication.

3. Research a case study of successful interdisciplinary collaboration in addressing food deserts. Summarize the findings and strategies employed by the research team. Discuss the importance of interdisciplinary collaboration in the context of the case study.

4. Consider the challenges mentioned in this section related to interdisciplinary collaboration. Propose strategies for overcoming these challenges in an interdisciplinary research project on food deserts. Justify your strategies based on the unique nature of food desert research.

5. Reflect on the benefits of interdisciplinary collaboration discussed in this section. Choose one benefit and explain how it can contribute to the development of comprehensive solutions for addressing food deserts. Provide a real-world example to support your explanation.

Key Takeaways

- Collaborative research across disciplines is essential for addressing complex issues like food deserts.

- Interdisciplinary collaboration provides diverse perspectives, creative problem-solving, synergistic teamwork, and comprehensive solutions.

- Challenges of interdisciplinary collaboration include communication barriers, power dynamics, time constraints, and methodological differences. These challenges can be addressed through effective strategies.

- Successful integration of interdisciplinary research involves establishing a common goal, building diverse teams, promoting effective communication, facilitating cross-disciplinary training, integrating methods, and emphasizing mutual respect and inclusion.

- Resources such as interdisciplinary journals, conferences, research centers, and grant programs can support interdisciplinary research on food deserts.

Further Reading

1. Roberts, P. (2017). *Interdisciplinarity and Food: Multiple Places of Engagements*. The Policy Press.

   This book explores the role of interdisciplinarity in understanding and addressing food-related issues, including food deserts. It provides insights into the challenges and benefits of interdisciplinary approaches and offers case studies from different contexts.

2. Ahern, M. M., Hendryx, M., & Roberts, M. J. (2019). Food deserts, access to food, and health behaviors among adults in Appalachia: Findings from a cross-sectional study. *BMC Public Health*, *19*(1), 1275.

   This article examines the relationship between food deserts, food access, and health behaviors in the context of Appalachia. It highlights the importance of interdisciplinary research in understanding the complexities of food deserts and their impact on health outcomes.

3. Coyle, K. (2016). *Food, Gender, and Poverty in the Ecuadorian Andes*. University of Pennsylvania Press.

   This book explores the intersection of food, gender, and poverty in the context of Ecuador and highlights the need for interdisciplinary approaches to understand the multifaceted nature of food inequalities.

4. Sallis, J. F., Cervero, R. B., Ascher, W., Henderson, K. A., Kraft, M. K., & Kerr, J. (2006). An ecological approach to creating active living communities. *Annual Review of Public Health, 27*, 297-322.

   This article presents an ecological approach to creating active living communities with a focus on urban design and transportation. It demonstrates the importance of interdisciplinary collaboration between urban planning, transportation, and public health disciplines to promote access to healthy food options.

Incorporating diverse perspectives and expertise

In order to fully understand and address the complex issue of food deserts, it is crucial to incorporate diverse perspectives and expertise. This not only enriches the research and interventions but also ensures a more comprehensive and inclusive approach. In this section, we will explore the importance of incorporating diverse perspectives and expertise in food desert research, and provide practical strategies for achieving this goal.

1. Importance of diverse perspectives: Food deserts are influenced by various factors such as socioeconomic status, race, ethnicity, geography, and culture. Each of these factors has unique implications for understanding and addressing the problem. By incorporating diverse perspectives, we can gain a more nuanced understanding of the different dimensions of food deserts and identify tailored solutions that consider and respect the needs and experiences of diverse communities.

2. The role of interdisciplinary collaboration: Food desert research requires a multidisciplinary approach as it encompasses various fields such as public health, urban planning, sociology, economics, geography, and nutrition. Each discipline brings its own theoretical framework, methodologies, and expertise. By collaborating across disciplines, researchers can benefit from different perspectives, methodologies, and research tools, leading to more comprehensive and robust findings.

3. Engaging community perspectives: Community engagement is a crucial component in addressing food deserts. Local residents have valuable knowledge and insights about their own communities, including culturally significant foods, barriers to access, and potential solutions. Involving community members in the research process not only ensures the relevance and effectiveness of interventions but also empowers communities to take ownership of their own well-being. Researchers can incorporate community perspectives through participatory research methods, community advisory boards, and partnerships with community-based organizations.

4. Inclusion of marginalized voices: Food deserts disproportionately affect marginalized populations such as low-income communities, racial and ethnic minorities, and immigrant populations. It is essential to center their experiences and voices in research and decision-making processes. Researchers can create a safe and inclusive environment for marginalized individuals to share their experiences, concerns, and aspirations. Additionally, conducting research with cultural humility and sensitivity ensures that interventions are respectful and tailored to the unique needs of marginalized populations.

5. Addressing implicit biases: Researchers must be mindful of their own implicit biases and recognize their potential impact on the research process and outcomes. Implicit biases can influence research questions, sampling methods, data interpretation, and interventions. Recognizing and addressing these biases is essential for conducting unbiased research and developing equitable interventions. Researchers can undergo training on implicit bias, incorporate diverse perspectives in research teams, and critically reflect on their own assumptions and perspectives.

6. Ethical considerations: Incorporating diverse perspectives and expertise requires a commitment to ethical research practices. This includes obtaining informed consent, protecting participant confidentiality, and ensuring research is conducted with integrity and respect for all involved. Researchers must also be aware of power imbalances and strive for equitable partnerships with community members, avoiding tokenism or exploitation.

By incorporating diverse perspectives and expertise, food desert research can generate knowledge that is more inclusive, equitable, and relevant. It allows for a deeper understanding of the complex factors contributing to food deserts and facilitates the development of interventions that address the specific needs and contexts of diverse communities. Ultimately, this approach can contribute to the creation of a more just and equitable food system.

Importance of interdisciplinary collaboration

Interdisciplinary collaboration plays a critical role in addressing the complex issue of food deserts. By bringing together experts from various fields, such as public health, urban planning, sociology, economics, and nutrition, we can gain a comprehensive understanding of the multifaceted nature of food deserts and develop effective solutions. In this section, we will explore the importance of interdisciplinary collaboration in food desert research and intervention efforts.

Understanding the Complexity of Food Deserts

Food deserts are not solely an issue of food access or geographic location. They are deeply intertwined with socioeconomic factors, health disparities, racial inequalities, and environmental justice. To effectively address food deserts, we need to consider the interconnectedness of these complex issues.

Collaboration between researchers and practitioners from diverse disciplines allows us to analyze food deserts from multiple perspectives and uncover the underlying causes and mechanisms. For example, economists can provide insights into the relationship between poverty and lack of healthy food options, while sociologists can shed light on the societal factors contributing to food deserts. This interdisciplinary approach enables us to develop a more nuanced understanding of the problem and identify effective intervention strategies.

Integration of Different Methodologies

Each discipline brings its unique methodologies and tools to the table, allowing us to gather comprehensive data and conduct robust analyses. Integrating quantitative and qualitative research methods leads to a more holistic understanding of food deserts.

Economists can employ statistical analyses to quantify the economic impacts of food deserts, such as the correlation between poverty rates and food access. Sociologists can conduct in-depth interviews and ethnographic studies to explore the lived experiences of individuals residing in food deserts and understand the social dynamics at play. By combining these different approaches, we can obtain a more accurate representation of the realities faced by communities affected by food deserts.

Identification of Synergies and Opportunities

Interdisciplinary collaboration also facilitates the identification of synergies and opportunities for innovative solutions. By bringing together experts with diverse perspectives, we can tap into their collective knowledge and unique skillsets to generate creative approaches.

For instance, urban planners can work with nutritionists to design community gardens and urban farms in food deserts, addressing both food access and environmental sustainability. Public health experts can collaborate with technological innovators to develop mobile apps that connect residents with local farmers markets and affordable, nutritious food options. These cross-discipline collaborations enable us to explore unconventional strategies that can have a transformative impact on food deserts.

Addressing Complex Challenges

Food deserts are complex problems that cannot be solved through a one-size-fits-all approach. The involvement of diverse disciplines ensures that we consider the underlying complexities and tailor interventions to the unique needs of each community.

Health disparities, food access, and poverty are deeply intertwined, requiring input from experts in different disciplines to develop comprehensive and sustainable solutions. Moreover, interdisciplinary collaboration helps us address the potential unintended consequences of interventions. For example, a policy aimed at increasing food access may inadvertently lead to gentrification or displacement if not carefully considered. By involving experts in urban planning and sociology, we can anticipate and mitigate such consequences.

Promoting Knowledge Transfer and Bridging Gaps

Interdisciplinary collaboration encourages knowledge transfer and the exchange of ideas between disciplines. Experts from different fields can learn from one another's perspectives, methodologies, and findings. This cross-pollination of ideas helps bridge gaps in understanding and can spark new research directions.

Furthermore, interdisciplinary collaboration fosters a more comprehensive and holistic approach to food desert research and interventions. It ensures that no important aspect or factor is overlooked by bringing together researchers who may have previously worked in isolation. The sharing of knowledge and expertise facilitates the development of comprehensive solutions that can have a meaningful impact on the lives of individuals living in food deserts.

Conclusion

In conclusion, interdisciplinary collaboration is crucial for addressing the challenges posed by food deserts. By combining the knowledge, skills, and perspectives of experts from various fields, we can develop a comprehensive understanding of the complex nature of food deserts and design effective strategies for intervention. Collaboration across disciplines enables us to approach the issue from multiple angles, integrate different methodologies, identify synergies, and address the inherent complexities. Moving forward, continued interdisciplinary collaboration will be essential for advancing research, policy development, and advocacy efforts to create lasting change and promote food justice in communities affected by food deserts.

Global Efforts to Address Food Deserts

International Policies and Strategies

International policies and strategies play a crucial role in addressing the issue of food deserts on a global scale. These policies aim to improve access to healthy and affordable food in underserved communities, promote sustainable food systems, and address the underlying causes of food deserts. In this section, we will explore some of the key international policies and strategies that have been implemented to tackle food deserts effectively.

The World Health Organization (WHO) Framework on Food Security

The World Health Organization (WHO) recognizes the importance of food security in promoting good health and well-being. The WHO framework on food security provides guidance and recommendations to governments and policymakers to address food deserts and ensure access to safe, nutritious, and culturally appropriate food for all individuals.

The framework emphasizes the need for a comprehensive approach to food security, which includes promoting sustainable agriculture, strengthening food distribution systems, improving infrastructure, and enhancing food governance. It also highlights the importance of addressing social determinants of health, such as poverty, inequality, and social exclusion, which are often closely linked to food deserts.

Furthermore, the WHO framework encourages countries to develop and implement multisectoral policies and strategies that involve various stakeholders, including governments, civil society organizations, and the private sector. Collaboration among these stakeholders is seen as essential for achieving sustainable solutions to food deserts.

The United Nations Sustainable Development Goals (SDGs)

The United Nations Sustainable Development Goals (SDGs) provide a global framework for addressing various social, economic, and environmental challenges, including food security and nutrition. SDG 2, specifically, focuses on achieving Zero Hunger and ensuring access to safe, nutritious, and sufficient food for all by 2030.

Under SDG 2, countries commit to implementing policies and interventions that promote sustainable agriculture, improve agricultural productivity, enhance the resilience of food production systems, and reduce post-harvest losses. These measures aim to address food deserts by increasing the availability and affordability of healthy food options, particularly for disadvantaged communities.

Additionally, the SDGs emphasize the importance of promoting sustainable food systems that minimize waste, conserve natural resources, and protect ecosystems. This approach recognizes the interconnectedness of food production, distribution, and consumption with environmental sustainability and underscores the need to tackle food deserts within the broader context of sustainability.

National Food Policies

Many countries around the world have developed their own national food policies to address food deserts and improve food security. These policies vary in their focus and strategies but generally aim to ensure access to healthy and affordable food for all individuals.

For example, the United Kingdom implemented the Healthy Food Financing Initiative, which provides financial support to increase the availability of healthy food retailers in underserved areas. The Scottish Government launched the Fair Food Transformation Fund, which supports community-led initiatives to tackle food poverty and promote food justice.

In the United States, the Healthy Food Financing Initiative was launched at the federal level to address food deserts and increase access to fresh and nutritious food in low-income communities. Many states and local governments have also implemented their own initiatives, such as offering tax incentives for grocery stores to establish in food desert areas.

International Partnerships and Collaborations

International partnerships and collaborations play a crucial role in addressing food deserts globally. Organizations such as the Food and Agriculture Organization of the United Nations (FAO), the United Nations Children's Fund (UNICEF), and the World Food Program (WFP) work together to develop and implement effective strategies to improve food security and access to nutritious food.

These organizations provide technical support, capacity building, and financial assistance to countries in need, particularly in low-income regions. They also facilitate knowledge sharing and promote best practices in addressing food deserts through conferences, workshops, and research publications.

Furthermore, international partnerships also involve collaborations with non-governmental organizations (NGOs), academic institutions, and private sector entities. These collaborations leverage diverse expertise and resources to develop innovative solutions and implement sustainable interventions in food deserts.

Examples of Successful International Policies and Strategies

Several countries have successfully implemented policies and strategies to address food deserts and improve food security. For instance, Brazil's National School Feeding Program (PNAE) ensures that all students have access to healthy and locally sourced meals in schools, thereby reducing food insecurity among children and promoting nutrition education.

In Canada, the Northern Healthy Food Program aims to improve access to healthy food in remote and isolated northern communities. The program provides funding and technical support for community-led initiatives, such as community gardens, greenhouse projects, and traditional food harvesting programs.

In Germany, the Federal Ministry of Food and Agriculture launched the "More Vegetables and Fruits in Schools and Kindergartens" initiative, which promotes the consumption of fruits and vegetables among children. The initiative includes education campaigns, school gardens, and partnerships with local farmers to ensure a steady supply of fresh produce.

These examples demonstrate the effectiveness of comprehensive policies and strategies in addressing food deserts and improving food security. They highlight the importance of involving multiple stakeholders, adopting a multisectoral approach, and tailoring interventions to the specific needs and contexts of communities.

Conclusion

In this section, we explored various international policies and strategies that have been implemented to tackle food deserts worldwide. These policies aim to improve access to healthy and affordable food, promote sustainable food systems, and address the underlying causes of food deserts.

The World Health Organization framework on food security provides guidance for governments to develop comprehensive strategies, while the United Nations Sustainable Development Goals emphasize the need for sustainable agriculture and food systems. National food policies and international collaborations further support efforts to address food deserts and achieve food security.

Successful examples from different countries illustrate the impact of these policies and strategies in improving food access and nutrition. However, challenges and limitations remain, necessitating ongoing research and advocacy to ensure equity and social justice in interventions. Future trends and interdisciplinary approaches will continue to shape the field of food desert research, enabling more effective and sustainable solutions for communities worldwide.

Transnational Partnerships and Collaborations

Transnational partnerships and collaborations play a crucial role in addressing food deserts globally. As the issue of food deserts extends beyond national boundaries, it requires a collective effort involving various stakeholders, including governments, non-profit organizations, research institutions, and community groups from different countries. This section examines the importance of transnational partnerships and collaborations in tackling food deserts, explores successful examples, and discusses the lessons learned from these initiatives.

Understanding the Importance of Transnational Partnerships

Transnational partnerships and collaborations offer several advantages in addressing food deserts. Firstly, they facilitate the exchange of knowledge, expertise, and best practices between countries. By sharing experiences and lessons learned, countries can avoid reinventing the wheel and instead build on successful initiatives implemented elsewhere.

Secondly, these partnerships enable pooling of resources, both financial and human, to implement comprehensive interventions. Food deserts require multidimensional solutions that involve infrastructural changes, policy reforms, educational programs, and community engagement. Transnational collaborations allow for a more holistic approach by leveraging the strengths and resources of multiple countries.

Thirdly, transnational partnerships provide a platform for advocacy and collective action. By uniting different countries around the common goal of addressing food deserts, there is a stronger voice to influence international policies, secure funding, and promote systemic changes.

Successful Examples of Transnational Partnerships

Several successful initiatives have demonstrated the positive impact of transnational partnerships and collaborations in addressing food deserts. Here are three notable examples:

1. **Scaling Up Nutrition (SUN)** SUN is a global movement that aims to address malnutrition, including food access issues, by bringing together governments, civil society organizations, businesses, and donors. The partnership currently includes 61 countries, working collectively to improve nutrition and reduce food insecurity. Through knowledge sharing and collaborative actions, SUN has been successful in implementing targeted interventions in various countries, including those affected by food deserts.

2. **Milan Urban Food Policy Pact** The Milan Urban Food Policy Pact is an international commitment signed by over 200 cities worldwide to develop sustainable food systems. Through this pact, cities collaborate to share innovative approaches, policies, and strategies to promote food security, including addressing food deserts. The pact facilitates knowledge transfer and encourages cities to learn from each other's experiences, enabling them to implement effective interventions tailored to their local context.

3. **Global Alliance for Improved Nutrition (GAIN)** GAIN is an international organization that works with governments, businesses, and civil society to improve nutrition and promote food security. Their focus includes addressing food deserts through partnerships across countries. GAIN collaborates with governments to develop policies, supports businesses in creating nutritious products, and engages communities to promote behavior change. The organization's transnational approach allows for cross-learning and sharing of successful strategies.

Lessons Learned and Challenges

While transnational partnerships offer great potential in addressing food deserts, they also face certain challenges. One key challenge is the variation in socio-economic and cultural contexts across countries. What works in one country may not be directly applicable in another due to differences in food systems, dietary preferences, and socio-economic disparities. Therefore, it is crucial to adapt interventions to local contexts while leveraging the learnings from other countries.

Another challenge is the need for sustained commitment and long-term funding. Food deserts are complex issues requiring multi-year interventions. Transnational partnerships must navigate the dynamics of funding and ensure a sustainable source of financial support for ongoing initiatives. This requires collaboration with international donors, philanthropic organizations, and governments to secure long-term funding commitments.

Additionally, effective communication and coordination among diverse stakeholders pose challenges. Overcoming language barriers, cultural differences, and power dynamics can be complex but necessary to ensure effective collaboration. Regular communication channels, clear roles and responsibilities, and inclusive decision-making processes are essential for successful transnational partnerships.

Conclusion

Transnational partnerships and collaborations are crucial in addressing food deserts globally. Through knowledge exchange, resource-sharing, and collective advocacy, these partnerships offer the potential to generate innovative solutions and create systemic change. Successful initiatives like the Scaling Up Nutrition movement, Milan Urban Food Policy Pact, and Global Alliance for Improved Nutrition demonstrate the positive impact of transnational collaborations.

However, challenges such as contextual differences, sustainable funding, and effective communication need to be addressed. By learning from successful examples and overcoming these challenges, transnational partnerships can play a significant role in achieving food justice and improving nutrition outcomes worldwide.

Exercises

1. Research and identify a transnational partnership or collaboration that has worked to address food deserts or a related issue. Present a case study outlining the initiative and its impact.

2. Discuss the potential benefits and challenges of transnational partnerships in addressing food deserts. Provide examples and draw from real-world experiences to support your arguments.

3. Imagine you are part of a team responsible for developing a transnational partnership to tackle food deserts. Outline the key steps you would take to establish and sustain this collaboration, considering the challenges and opportunities involved.

4. Conduct a comparative analysis of food deserts in two different countries. Discuss the similarities and differences in their underlying causes, impacts, and existing interventions. Identify potential areas for transnational collaboration and propose innovative solutions based on the comparative analysis.

5. Explore the role of technology in facilitating transnational partnerships. Investigate how digital platforms and online tools can bridge the gap between different countries working towards addressing food deserts.

Further Reading

1. United Nations [website]. Scaling Up Nutrition (SUN) Movement. Available at: `https://scalingupnutrition.org/` 2. Milan Urban Food Policy Pact [website]. Available at: `https://www.milanurbanfoodpolicypact.org/` 3. Global Alliance for Improved Nutrition [website]. Available at: `https://www.gainhealth.org/` 4. Clancy, K. (2017). Transnational Urbanism and the Food Sovereignty Movement. Journal of Urban Affairs, 39(4), 461-478. 5. Neefjes, K. (2019). Concrete steps towards city-led global good governance: The Milan Urban Food Policy Pact. World Development, 122, 598-607.

Lessons learned from other countries

When examining the issue of food deserts, it is important to consider the experiences and lessons learned from other countries around the world. By studying different approaches and strategies employed in various contexts, we can gain valuable insights and identify best practices that can inform our efforts in addressing food deserts.

One country that has made significant progress in combating food deserts is the United Kingdom. The British government has taken a holistic approach, focusing on both policy and community-based interventions. One notable policy is the Healthy Start program, which provides vouchers to low-income families to purchase fresh fruits, vegetables, and milk. This initiative has not only improved access to nutritious foods but also enhanced the financial well-being of vulnerable households. Additionally, the UK has implemented zoning regulations that limit the concentration of fast food outlets in areas with high levels of deprivation.

Another country that has successfully tackled the issue of food deserts is Australia. The Australian government has prioritized the promotion of healthy food retail in underserved areas through initiatives such as the Healthy Food Access Basket program. This program involves engaging local retailers to stock and promote healthier food options, addressing issues of affordability and availability. Furthermore, Australia has invested in community-led initiatives such as community gardens and farmers markets to foster community ownership and engagement in improving food access.

In Japan, the concept of "satoyama" has been instrumental in addressing food deserts. Satoyama refers to the sustainable management of forested rural landscapes, incorporating agricultural practices that provide fresh and diverse food sources for local communities. By integrating agriculture, forestry, and fisheries, Japan has been able to ensure the availability of nutritious foods in both urban and rural areas. Additionally, the Japanese government has implemented policies that support small-scale farmers and enhance local food systems, further contributing to food security and reducing food deserts.

Lessons can also be learned from South Africa, where the concept of "food sovereignty" has gained prominence. Food sovereignty emphasizes the rights of communities to control their own food systems and make decisions about the production, distribution, and consumption of food. In South Africa, initiatives such as urban agriculture projects, community food gardens, and mobile markets have been successful in reducing food deserts and empowering communities to take ownership of their food security. These efforts have demonstrated the importance of community participation and empowerment in achieving sustainable solutions.

It is important to note that while lessons from other countries can provide valuable insights, there is no one-size-fits-all solution to addressing food deserts. Context-specific factors such as cultural norms, institutional frameworks, and socioeconomic conditions must be considered when implementing interventions. Additionally, ongoing evaluation and monitoring of interventions are crucial to understand their effectiveness and ensure long-term sustainability.

In conclusion, studying the experiences of other countries can offer valuable lessons and best practices in addressing food deserts. Initiatives and policies from the United Kingdom, Australia, Japan, and South Africa provide insights into effective strategies such as government-led programs, community-based approaches, sustainable agricultural practices, and prioritizing community empowerment. By learning from these experiences and tailoring interventions to specific contexts, we can work towards achieving equitable and sustainable access to healthy food for all.

The Role of Advocacy and Activism

Grassroots movements and community organizing

Grassroots movements and community organizing play a crucial role in addressing food deserts and advocating for food justice. These efforts are driven by community members who mobilize to create change and improve access to healthy and affordable food. In this section, we will explore the principles, strategies, and impact of grassroots movements and community organizing in the context of food deserts.

Principles of Grassroots Movements

Grassroots movements are driven by the collective power of individuals within a community. They are generally focused on addressing social, economic, or environmental injustices. In the case of food deserts, grassroots movements seek to dismantle the systemic barriers that contribute to limited food access. The following principles guide grassroots movements:

1. Empowerment: Grassroots movements operate under the belief that communities have the knowledge, expertise, and agency to address their own issues. They empower individuals to take the lead in creating change and advocate for their own needs.
2. Inclusivity: Grassroots movements aim to involve diverse individuals and groups within a community. They prioritize inclusivity to ensure that the voices of marginalized populations are heard and represented in decision-making processes.
3. Collaboration: Grassroots movements often work through collaborative efforts, bringing together various stakeholders, such as community members, local organizations, and activists, to maximize their impact. Collaboration fosters a sense of solidarity and strengthens the movement's ability to enact change.
4. Grassroots Leadership: Grassroots movements are driven by leaders who emerge from within the community. These leaders possess a deep understanding of the local context and have earned the trust and respect of their community members.

Strategies for Community Organizing

Community organizing is a key strategy employed by grassroots movements to address food deserts. It involves mobilizing community members, raising awareness, and advocating for policy changes. Here are some effective strategies for community organizing in the context of food deserts:

1. Building Relationships: Successful community organizing begins with building relationships within the community. Organizers engage with community members, listen to their concerns, and establish trust. These relationships serve as a foundation for collective action.

2. Education and Awareness: Community organizing efforts focus on educating community members about the impact of food deserts on their health and well-being. By raising awareness, organizers empower individuals to make informed choices and take action.

3. Community Surveys and Mapping: Conducting community surveys and mapping exercises helps identify the specific needs and challenges of a community. This data provides valuable insights for organizing efforts and strengthens the case for policy change.

4. Advocacy and Policy Reform: Organizers engage in advocacy at the local, regional, and national levels to push for policy reforms that improve food access. They collaborate with policymakers, attend public meetings, and make their voices heard to drive change.

5. Direct Action and Grassroots Initiatives: Grassroots movements often employ direct action tactics, such as protests, marches, and boycotts, to draw attention to food deserts and demand immediate action. Additionally, organizing initiatives, such as community gardens, farmers markets, and food cooperatives, provide practical solutions that increase access to fresh and healthy food.

Case Studies of Successful Grassroots Movements

There have been several successful grassroots movements that have made a significant impact in addressing food deserts. Let's explore a few notable case studies:

1. The Detroit Black Community Food Security Network: This grassroots organization was established in response to the lack of access to fresh food in Detroit's predominantly Black neighborhoods. They initiated several community-based projects, including urban farms, farmers markets, and a food buying club, to increase access to healthy food and educate the community about sustainable food systems.

2. The Camden Food Co-op: In Camden, New Jersey, community organizers established a cooperative grocery store to combat food deserts. The co-op operates on the principles of democratic ownership and prioritizes sourcing fresh and local produce. Through collective ownership, the co-op provides affordable and nutritious food options to an underserved community.

3. The Navajo Nation Community Food Sovereignty Initiative: The Navajo Nation, located in the southwestern United States, faces significant food access challenges due to its remote location and historical marginalization. Grassroots organizing efforts have focused on revitalizing traditional food systems, supporting local farmers, and promoting sustainable agriculture. These initiatives work to restore food sovereignty and improve access to cultural and nutritious foods within the Navajo Nation.

Challenges and Tips for Grassroots Movements

While grassroots movements hold significant potential for addressing food deserts, they also face several challenges. Here are some common challenges and tips for overcoming them:

1. Resource Constraints: Grassroots movements often operate with limited financial resources. Seeking partnerships, applying for grants, and engaging in fundraising efforts can help secure the necessary resources to sustain organizing initiatives.

2. Sustained Engagement: Maintaining community engagement and sustaining momentum over time can be challenging. To address this, organizers should prioritize building long-term relationships, regularly communicate with the community, and celebrate small wins along the way.

3. Overcoming Resistance: Grassroots movements may face resistance from powerful actors or entrenched systems. Building coalitions, leveraging media attention, and employing strategic communication can help overcome resistance and amplify the movement's message.

4. Intersectionality and Inclusivity: Addressing the intersectional nature of food justice ensures that the needs of all community members are met. Grassroots movements should actively work to include diverse voices, actively listen to marginalized communities, and prioritize equity in decision-making processes.

In conclusion, grassroots movements and community organizing play a vital role in addressing food deserts and advocating for food justice. Through empowerment, collaboration, and strategic action, grassroots movements mobilize communities, raise awareness, and drive policy changes. Despite challenges, successful grassroots movements have proven that change is possible when individuals come together to demand equitable access to healthy and affordable food.

Influencing Policy and Structural Change

In order to effectively address the issue of food deserts and promote food justice, it is crucial to advocate for policy and structural changes at the local, regional, and national levels. This section explores various strategies and approaches that can be employed to influence policy and bring about transformative change.

Understanding the Role of Advocacy

Advocacy plays a significant role in raising awareness about the challenges faced by communities living in food deserts and advocating for appropriate policy interventions. Advocacy efforts can range from grassroots movements to community organizing and lobbying government officials. By amplifying the voices of affected individuals and communities, advocates can drive systemic change and push for policies that address food inequality in a comprehensive and sustainable manner.

It is important for advocates to understand the power dynamics at play and be well-versed in the social, political, and economic factors that contribute to the existence of food deserts. By analyzing these structural inequities, advocates can effectively identify areas where policy changes are most needed and develop targeted strategies to influence decision-makers.

Collaboration and Coalition Building

Influencing policy and structural change requires building coalitions and collaborating with diverse stakeholders, including community organizations, non-profit organizations, researchers, policymakers, and businesses. These collaborations can help to leverage resources, expertise, and networks to drive meaningful change.

By working together, advocates can pool their knowledge, skills, and resources to develop policy recommendations, draft legislation, and undertake advocacy campaigns. Moreover, building coalitions allows for the creation of a collective voice, which reinforces the urgency and importance of addressing food deserts as a social justice issue.

Policy Research and Analysis

Evidence-based research and analysis are critical to informing policy debates and shaping solutions that address the root causes of food deserts. Advocates can contribute to policy discussions by conducting research studies, analyzing existing data, and producing reports that highlight the impact of food deserts on community health, economic development, and social well-being.

Through research, advocates can identify successful interventions and best practices from other regions or countries, demonstrating the feasibility and potential impact of specific policy measures. This evidence can be used to make convincing arguments to policymakers, providing them with the necessary information and data to support policy changes.

Policy Proposals and Recommendations

Advocates can develop policy proposals and recommendations that aim to address the structural barriers contributing to food deserts. These proposals should be comprehensive and multifaceted, considering the economic, social, and environmental dimensions of food access.

Policy recommendations may include:

1. Increased funding for the development of grocery stores, farmers markets, and other food retail outlets in underserved areas. 2. Zoning and land-use policies that prioritize the establishment of healthy food outlets in food desert regions. 3. Financial incentives or tax breaks for businesses that invest in underserved communities. 4. Transportation policies that improve access to healthy food options, such as expanded public transportation services or subsidized transportation programs. 5. Support for urban agriculture and community gardening initiatives through zoning changes, technical assistance, and funding. 6. Integration of food access and nutrition education into school curricula and community programs.

Engaging Decision-Makers

To influence policy and structural change, advocates must engage decision-makers at various levels, including local, state, and federal governments. This can be achieved through direct engagement, such as meeting with elected officials, participating in public hearings, and submitting written testimony. Additionally, advocates can utilize digital platforms and social media to raise awareness, share stories, and garner public support for policy initiatives.

It is crucial for advocates to clearly articulate the impact of food deserts on community health, economic vitality, and social well-being. By illustrating the connections between food access, nutrition, education, employment, and other key issues, advocates can make a compelling case for policy change. Moreover, building relationships with decision-makers and establishing trust can enhance the credibility and effectiveness of advocacy efforts.

Addressing Power Structures and Inequities

Influencing policy and structural change requires challenging power structures and addressing systemic inequities that perpetuate food deserts. This involves advocating for social justice and equity in decision-making processes, as well as dismantling barriers that prevent marginalized communities from actively participating in shaping policies that affect their lives.

Advocates can work towards addressing power imbalances by promoting inclusive and participatory decision-making processes. This can include working with community members to develop their leadership skills, providing them with the necessary tools and resources to engage in policy discussions, and advocating for the representation of diverse voices in decision-making bodies.

Monitoring and Evaluation

To ensure the effectiveness of policy and structural changes, continuous monitoring and evaluation are essential. Advocates can play a key role in monitoring the implementation of policies, tracking progress, and assessing their impact on food access and community well-being.

By collecting and analyzing relevant data, advocates can hold policymakers accountable and advocate for necessary adjustments or improvements to existing policies. Monitoring and evaluation can also help identify challenges and barriers that may arise during the implementation phase and inform future policy advocacy efforts.

Conclusion

Influencing policy and structural change is a crucial component of addressing food deserts and promoting food justice. Through advocacy, collaboration, and evidence-based research, advocates can advance policy proposals, engage decision-makers, and challenge power structures to create sustainable solutions that address the root causes of food deserts.

By actively participating in policy debates, raising awareness, and mobilizing communities, advocates can bring about transformative change that improves food access, promotes health equity, and builds a more just and inclusive food system. It is through collective action and advocacy that we can create a future where everyone has equitable access to nutritious and affordable food.

Building a Collective Voice for Food Justice

In order to effectively address food deserts and advocate for systemic change, building a collective voice for food justice is crucial. This section explores the power of advocacy and activism in creating positive social impact and offers strategies for individuals and communities to amplify their voices.

The Importance of Advocacy

Advocacy plays a crucial role in promoting equity and social justice in relation to food access. It involves raising awareness, engaging the public, and influencing policymakers to take action. By advocating for food justice, individuals and communities can work towards creating a more inclusive and equitable food system.

Grassroots Movements and Community Organizing

Grassroots movements and community organizing are key components of building a collective voice for food justice. These efforts start at the local level and empower individuals and communities to take action. Grassroots movements often focus on mobilizing community members, organizing protests, raising public awareness, and demanding policy changes.

Community organizing, on the other hand, involves bringing people together, identifying shared goals, and initiating collective actions. It provides a platform for individuals and groups to collaborate and address food access issues within their communities. Through grassroots movements and community organizing, people can exert their influence and bring attention to the problems faced by marginalized communities in food deserts.

Influencing Policy and Structural Change

Advocacy for food justice involves influencing policy and structural change to address underlying causes of food deserts. Policies play a critical role in shaping food systems, and advocating for policy changes is essential for combating food inequality.

One effective strategy for influencing policy is through lobbying. Lobbying involves engaging with elected officials and policymakers to promote specific policy reforms. By sharing personal stories, providing evidence-based research, and partnering with like-minded organizations, individuals and communities can effectively advocate for policy changes that address food access issues.

Furthermore, building relationships and coalitions with other stakeholders, such as community organizations, businesses, and academic institutions, can enhance the collective voice for food justice. These collaborations can amplify the impact of advocacy efforts and help drive systemic change.

Building a Collective Voice

To build a collective voice for food justice, it is important to create spaces for dialogue and collaboration. This can be achieved through community forums, town hall meetings, and online platforms. These platforms provide opportunities for individuals and communities to share their experiences, exchange ideas, and develop collective strategies for addressing food deserts.

Additionally, building alliances with existing social justice movements can amplify the voice of food justice advocates. By connecting with organizations working on issues such as racial justice, income inequality, and environmental justice, the collective voice for food justice can gain strength and visibility.

Promoting Public Awareness

Generating public awareness is crucial for building a collective voice for food justice. It involves disseminating information, raising consciousness about food deserts and their impacts, and mobilizing public support for change. Public awareness campaigns can leverage various communication channels, such as social media, traditional media, and community events, to educate the public and inspire action.

Moreover, storytelling and personal narratives have tremendous power in engaging the public and conveying the lived experiences of individuals affected by food deserts. Sharing stories of resilience, community-led initiatives, and the impacts of food justice interventions can inspire empathy and galvanize support.

Capacity Building and Leadership Development

Building a collective voice for food justice requires capacity building and leadership development within communities. Providing education and resources to community members empowers them to advocate for change effectively. Workshops, training programs, and mentorship opportunities can equip individuals with the skills and knowledge needed to engage in advocacy efforts.

Furthermore, nurturing grassroots leaders and providing them with platforms for leadership can strengthen the collective voice for food justice. Leadership development programs can cultivate a diverse set of leaders, ensuring that the movement reflects the perspectives and experiences of the communities affected by food deserts.

Measuring Impact and Celebrating Success

Measuring the impact of advocacy efforts is essential for assessing progress and refining strategies. Tracking policy changes, improvements in food access, and positive health outcomes can demonstrate the effectiveness of advocacy initiatives. This data can be used to celebrate successes and inspire continued action.

Additionally, recognizing and celebrating the achievements of individuals, community organizations, and movements involved in food justice advocacy can build momentum and strengthen solidarity. Award ceremonies, community events, and media coverage can acknowledge the contributions made towards building a collective voice for food justice.

Conclusion

Building a collective voice for food justice is a critical component of addressing food deserts and promoting social change. Through grassroots movements, community organizing, advocacy efforts, and collaborations, individuals and communities can amplify their voices and advocate for policies and structural changes that address food access disparities. By promoting public awareness, capacity building, and leadership development, and measuring impact, the collective voice for food justice can create a more equitable and inclusive food system.

Conclusion

Conclusion

Recap of Key Findings and Takeaways

Throughout this book, we have explored the concept of food deserts and the profound impact they have on nutrition and health inequalities. In this final section, let us recap the key findings and takeaways from our investigation.

1. Food deserts are defined as areas with limited access to affordable and nutritious food, often due to the absence of grocery stores or other fresh food retailers. Factors contributing to the emergence of food deserts include low income levels, transportation barriers, educational attainment, employment opportunities, and racial disparities.

2. The geographical distribution of food deserts in the United States is a significant issue, with both urban and rural areas affected. Demographic characteristics such as race, ethnicity, and socioeconomic status play a crucial role in determining the prevalence of food deserts.

3. Internationally, food deserts exist in different countries, demonstrating global trends and challenges. Case studies from various nations reveal commonalities and differences in the underlying causes and potential solutions to address food deserts.

4. Various theoretical frameworks help us understand the complexity of food deserts. Socioeconomic theories highlight the role of poverty and income disparities in determining food access. Health disparities and food justice frameworks emphasize the importance of equitable food distribution and the impact of food deserts on public health.

5. Socioeconomic factors, such as poverty and economic inequality, significantly influence the prevalence of food deserts. Higher poverty rates and income disparities are associated with limited access to healthy food options and higher rates of food insecurity.

6. Access to transportation is a vital determinant of food access in food deserts. Transportation barriers, especially in low-income communities, limit individuals' ability to travel to grocery stores or supermarkets. Innovative solutions, including public transportation and community-based transportation programs, can help overcome these challenges.

7. Education plays a critical role in shaping food choices and nutritional knowledge. Higher educational attainment is associated with better nutrition practices and healthier food preferences. Addressing the education gap in food deserts is essential for improving overall nutrition and health literacy.

8. Employment opportunities in food deserts are often limited, leading to income instability and food insecurity. Government assistance programs, such as Supplemental Nutrition Assistance Program (SNAP), play a crucial role in supporting individuals and families in accessing affordable and nutritious food.

9. Racial and ethnic disparities persist in food access, with minority communities facing higher rates of food deserts. Historical and socio-cultural factors contribute to these inequalities, and addressing systemic racism is necessary to achieve equitable food access.

10. Food deserts have significant health impacts, including nutritional deficiencies, increased risk of obesity, and the development of chronic diseases. Additionally, food insecurity in food deserts has detrimental effects on mental health, childhood development, environmental health, and healthy aging.

In addressing food deserts, an array of solutions and interventions has been explored throughout this book:

11. Policy changes and government initiatives have been implemented to combat food deserts. Legislation has been enacted to incentivize grocery store development in underserved areas, and government-funded programs have focused on increasing access to healthy food options.

12. Community-based approaches, such as community gardens and farmers markets, have emerged as successful strategies to improve food access in food deserts. These initiatives foster community engagement, empower local residents, and promote sustainable and locally sourced food options.

13. Technological solutions like mobile apps and online platforms have the potential to bridge the food access gap in food deserts. Food delivery services specifically designed for underserved areas have shown promise in improving accessibility to fresh and healthy food.

14. Education and health promotion efforts are crucial for addressing the knowledge gap regarding nutrition and health in food deserts. Nutrition education programs in schools and communities, coupled with public health campaigns, can empower individuals with the necessary knowledge to make healthier food choices.

15. Non-profit organizations and philanthropic efforts play a vital role in addressing food deserts through funding, support, and community partnerships. Building collaborations among stakeholders is essential for sustainable and impactful interventions.

As we evaluate the impact of interventions, it is vital to:

16. Develop effective methods for measuring the success of interventions, including monitoring food access, health outcomes, and social and economic indicators of progress.

17. Highlight case studies of successful interventions, analyzing the factors contributing to their efficacy and applicability.

18. Recognize the challenges and limitations of interventions, addressing systemic barriers and focusing on long-term sustainability. Learning from unsuccessful interventions is equally critical in refining our approach to addressing food deserts.

19. Emphasize equity and social justice in intervention strategies, ensuring that interventions do not perpetuate existing inequalities but rather prioritize the inclusion and empowerment of marginalized communities.

Looking towards the future, several trends and directions in food desert research emerge:

20. The impact of climate change on food deserts requires attention, as changing environmental conditions can exacerbate the challenges already faced by underserved communities.

21. The COVID-19 pandemic has further highlighted the vulnerabilities of food deserts, making it necessary to analyze the specific effects of the pandemic on food access and develop strategies to mitigate its impact.

22. Innovative solutions, such as vertical farming and hydroponics, hold promise for addressing food deserts effectively.

23. Interdisciplinary collaboration is essential for comprehensive and holistic research on food deserts. Collaborative efforts across disciplines enable a broader understanding of the multifaceted nature of this complex issue.

24. Global efforts to address food deserts provide valuable insights and lessons that can be adapted and implemented in different contexts.

25. Advocacy and activism play a vital role in bringing about structural change and promoting social justice in relation to food access. Grassroots movements and community organizing can influence policy and create a collective voice for food justice.

In conclusion, addressing food deserts requires a multifaceted approach encompassing policy changes, community-based initiatives, technological innovations, education, and collaboration. By understanding the causes, consequences, and potential solutions to food deserts, we can work towards achieving equitable access to healthy and nutritious food for all. Let us embark on this journey together, advocating for lasting change and fostering a more just and inclusive food system.

Call to Action for Addressing Food Deserts

Addressing the issue of food deserts requires a collective effort from various stakeholders, including policymakers, community leaders, non-profit organizations, and individuals. While the complexities surrounding food deserts may seem daunting, there are tangible steps that can be taken to mitigate the problem and promote food justice. This section provides a call to action, outlining key strategies and recommendations to address food deserts effectively.

Policy Changes and Government Initiatives

One crucial step in addressing food deserts is the implementation of policy changes and government initiatives. Policymakers can play a significant role in creating an enabling environment that fosters equitable food access. Some key strategies and recommendations include:

- **Legislation addressing food deserts:** Governments can enact laws that incentivize the establishment of grocery stores and fresh food markets in underserved areas. This can be done through tax credits, grants, or zoning regulations that prioritize food access.

- **Government-funded programs and initiatives:** Governments at all levels can allocate funding to support initiatives aimed at reducing food deserts. This can include financial support for community gardens, farmers markets, and transportation programs that improve access to healthy food options.

- **Evaluation of policy effectiveness:** Regular evaluation and monitoring of policy interventions are crucial to ensure their effectiveness. Governments should invest in data collection and analysis to assess the impact of policy changes on food access and nutrition outcomes.

Community-Based Approaches

Community-based approaches play a vital role in addressing food deserts, as they empower individuals and foster a sense of collective responsibility. Some strategies and recommendations for community-based interventions include:

- **Community gardens and urban farming:** Encouraging the establishment of community gardens and urban farming initiatives can provide local residents with access to fresh produce and the knowledge and skills needed for sustainable food production.

- **Farmers markets and food cooperatives:** Support for farmers markets and food cooperatives can contribute to food access by providing affordable and locally sourced products. These initiatives also create economic opportunities for local farmers and producers.

- **Collaborative efforts and community empowerment:** Building partnerships between community organizations, non-profit groups, and local government can lead to collective action and community empowerment. Collaborative efforts can include advocacy campaigns, education programs, and resource-sharing initiatives.

Technological Solutions

In the digital age, technology can serve as a powerful tool for addressing food deserts. Technological solutions can help bridge gaps in food access and facilitate efficient delivery systems. Some strategies and recommendations for leveraging technology to address food deserts include:

- **Mobile apps and online platforms:** Developing mobile applications and online platforms can provide information on nearby food resources, including grocery stores, farmers markets, and food assistance programs. These tools can also facilitate direct ordering and delivery of fresh produce and healthy food options.

- **Food delivery services in food deserts:** Collaborating with existing food delivery services to ensure coverage of food deserts can provide convenient access to nutritious food, especially for individuals without reliable transportation or limited mobility.

- **Using technology to bridge the food access gap:** Innovative approaches, such as using drones or autonomous vehicles for food delivery, can help overcome transportation barriers and ensure timely and reliable access to healthy food options.

Education and Health Promotion

Education and health promotion efforts are critical components of addressing food deserts. By empowering individuals with nutrition knowledge and promoting healthy behaviors, long-term changes in food access and food choices can be achieved. Some strategies and recommendations for education and health promotion include:

- **Nutrition education in schools and communities:** Integrating nutrition education into school curricula and community programs can equip individuals with the knowledge and skills necessary to make informed food choices and advocate for healthier food environments.
- **Public health campaigns in food deserts:** Engaging with communities through targeted public health campaigns can raise awareness about the importance of healthy eating and the impact of food deserts. These campaigns should provide practical information and resources to support behavior change.
- **Empowering individuals with nutrition knowledge:** Providing accessible and culturally appropriate information about nutrition and healthy food choices can empower individuals to navigate food deserts and make informed decisions about their diets.

Non-Profit Organizations and Philanthropic Efforts

Non-profit organizations and philanthropic initiatives play a crucial role in addressing food deserts, as they often have the flexibility and expertise to implement innovative solutions. Some strategies and recommendations for non-profit organizations and philanthropic efforts include:

- **Initiatives by non-profit organizations:** Non-profit organizations can lead the way in developing and implementing interventions that target food deserts, such as community gardening programs, mobile food markets, and nutrition education initiatives.
- **Funding and support for food desert interventions:** Philanthropic organizations can provide financial support and resources to community-driven projects that aim to address food deserts. This support can be in the form of grants, technical assistance, capacity-building, and research funding.

- **Building partnerships and collaborations:** Non-profit organizations and philanthropic entities should prioritize building partnerships and collaborations with community organizations, government agencies, and academic institutions. These collaborations can help leverage resources, share best practices, and promote sustainable solutions.

In conclusion, addressing food deserts requires a multifaceted approach that combines policy changes, community-based initiatives, technological solutions, education, and non-profit efforts. By implementing the strategies and recommendations outlined in this section, we can work towards creating equitable access to healthy food, promoting food justice, and mitigating the adverse effects of food deserts on communities. Collectively, we have the power to make a difference and ensure that everyone has the opportunity to thrive with adequate nutrition.

Future Directions in Food Desert Research

The study of food deserts is an ever-evolving field that requires ongoing research and investigation. As we continue to address the complex issues surrounding food inequality and access, several avenues of future research have emerged. In this section, we will explore some of these promising directions and highlight the areas where further investigation is needed.

Understanding the Impact of Climate Change

One important area for future research is the impact of climate change on food deserts. With global warming and environmental degradation, there is a growing concern about how these factors will exacerbate the problem of food inequality. Rising temperatures, changes in precipitation patterns, and extreme weather events can disrupt food production and distribution systems, particularly in already vulnerable areas.

Further research is needed to understand how climate change will affect the prevalence and severity of food deserts. This includes studying the potential impact on crop yields, food availability, and the ability of communities to access nutritious options. Additionally, exploring strategies for adapting to and mitigating the effects of climate change in food desert areas is crucial.

Effects of COVID-19 on Food Access

The COVID-19 pandemic has highlighted and exacerbated existing disparities in food access. The closure of businesses, disruptions in the supply chain, and economic hardships have disproportionately affected low-income communities, further deepening food insecurity.

Future research should focus on understanding the short-term and long-term effects of the pandemic on food deserts. This includes evaluating the effectiveness of emergency food distribution programs, the impact of school closures on children's access to nutritious meals, and the resilience of local food systems during times of crisis. Additionally, studying the ways in which communities mobilize and adapt to meet the challenges of food access during a pandemic can provide valuable insights for future interventions.

Innovative Solutions for the Future

As technology continues to advance, there is a growing potential for innovative solutions to address food deserts. Future research should explore the role of emerging technologies such as artificial intelligence, blockchain, and mobile applications in improving food access and reducing inequalities.

For example, artificial intelligence can be used to develop optimized food distribution systems that consider factors such as transportation logistics, demand forecasting, and community preferences. Blockchain technology can enhance transparency and traceability in the food supply chain, ensuring fair and equitable access to nutritious options. Mobile applications can provide real-time information about food availability, discounts, and cooking tips, empowering individuals to make healthier choices.

Furthermore, exploring the potential of vertical farming, aquaponics, and other sustainable agricultural practices can contribute to increasing local food production and reducing dependency on external food sources. Research in these areas can provide valuable insights into the feasibility and scalability of these solutions in food desert environments.

Interdisciplinary Collaboration

Given the complex nature of food deserts, future research should embrace interdisciplinary collaboration. Bringing together experts from various fields such as public health, urban planning, sociology, economics, and environmental science can enrich our understanding of the multifaceted factors influencing food inequality.

By combining diverse perspectives and expertise, researchers can develop comprehensive and holistic approaches to address food deserts. This includes exploring the social, economic, and environmental determinants of food access, evaluating the impact of interventions from multiple angles, and identifying potential synergies between different disciplines.

Global Efforts and Cross-Cultural Understanding

While much of the existing research on food deserts has focused on the United States, future studies should expand their scope to include a global perspective. Understanding food desert trends and interventions in different countries can provide valuable insights and lessons for addressing food inequality across diverse cultural and socioeconomic contexts.

Research should also explore the impact of globalization and trade policies on food access, taking into account the relationship between developed and developing nations. By examining cross-cultural variations in food deserts and analyzing the effectiveness of international policies and strategies, we can foster global collaborations and knowledge exchange in the fight against food inequality.

Advocacy, Activism, and Structural Change

Finally, future research should explore the role of advocacy and activism in addressing food deserts. Grassroots movements, community organizing, and policy advocacy have been instrumental in raising awareness about food inequality and driving change. Understanding the strategies, successes, and challenges of these efforts can inform future interventions and policy recommendations.

Research should also examine the structural and systemic barriers that perpetuate food deserts, including issues of power, privilege, and inequality. By identifying and addressing these root causes, we can work towards creating more just and equitable food systems for all.

In conclusion, future research in the field of food desert studies should focus on understanding the impact of climate change, investigating the effects of the COVID-19 pandemic, exploring innovative technological solutions, embracing interdisciplinary collaboration, expanding the global perspective, and examining the role of advocacy and activism. By pursuing these avenues, we can work towards more comprehensive and effective strategies for addressing food inequality and creating healthier, more equitable communities.

% Index

Index

9 781778 904868

Printed by Libri Plureos GmbH in Hamburg,
Germany